T0264199

Sexual Deviation: Assessment and Treatment

Editors

JOHN M.W. BRADFORD
A.G. AHMED

PSYCHIATRIC CLINICS OF NORTH AMERICA

www.psych.theclinics.com

June 2014 • Volume 37 • Number 2

ELSEVIER

1600 John F. Kennedy Boulevard • Suite 1800 • Philadelphia, Pennsylvania, 19103-2899

http://www.theclinics.com

PSYCHIATRIC CLINICS OF NORTH AMERICA Volume 37, Number 2
June 2014 ISSN 0193-953X, ISBN-13: 978-0-323-29931-2

Editor: Joanne Husovski
Developmental Editor: Stephanie Carter

© **2014 Elsevier Inc. All rights reserved.**

This periodical and the individual contributions contained in it are protected under copyright by Elsevier, and the following terms and conditions apply to their use:

Photocopying
Single photocopies of single articles may be made for personal use as allowed by national copyright laws. Permission of the Publisher and payment of a fee is required for all other photocopying, including multiple or systematic copying, copying for advertising or promotional purposes, resale, and all forms of document delivery. Special rates are available for educational institutions that wish to make photocopies for non-profit educational classroom use. For information on how to seek permission visit www.elsevier.com/permissions or call: (+44) 1865 843830 (UK)/(+1) 215 239 3804 (USA).

Derivative Works
Subscribers may reproduce tables of contents or prepare lists of articles including abstracts for internal circulation within their institutions. Permission of the Publisher is required for resale or distribution outside the institution. Permission of the Publisher is required for all other derivative works, including compilations and translations (please consult www.elsevier.com/permissions).

Electronic Storage or Usage
Permission of the Publisher is required to store or use electronically any material contained in this periodical, including any article or part of an article (please consult www.elsevier.com/permissions). Except as outlined above, no part of this publication may be reproduced, stored in a retrieval system or transmitted in any form or by any means, electronic, mechanical, photocopying, recording or otherwise, without prior written permission of the Publisher.

Notice
No responsibility is assumed by the Publisher for any injury and/or damage to persons or property as a matter of products liability, negligence or otherwise, or from any use or operation of any methods, products, instructions or ideas contained in the material herein. Because of rapid advances in the medical sciences, in particular, independent verification of diagnoses and drug dosages should be made.

Although all advertising material is expected to conform to ethical (medical) standards, inclusion in this publication does not constitute a guarantee or endorsement of the quality or value of such product or of the claims made of it by its manufacturer.

Psychiatric Clinics of North America (ISSN 0193-953X) is published quarterly by Elsevier Inc., 360 Park Avenue South, New York, NY 10010-1710. Months of issue are March, June, September, and December. Business and Editorial Offices: 1600 John F. Kennedy Blvd., Suite 1800, Philadelphia, PA 19103-2899. Periodicals postage paid at New York, NY and additional mailing offices. Subscription prices are $300.00 per year (US individuals), $546.00 per year (US institutions), $150.00 per year (US students/residents), $365.00 per year (Canadian individuals), $687.00 per year (Canadian Institutions), $455.00 per year (foreign individuals), $687.00 per year (foreign institutions), and $220.00 per year (international & Canadian students/residents). Foreign air speed delivery is included in all *Clinics'* subscription prices. All prices are subject to change without notice. **POSTMASTER:** Send address changes to *Psychiatric Clinics of North America*, Elsevier Health Sciences Division, Subscription Customer Service, 3251 Riverport Lane, Maryland Heights, MO 63043. Customer Service: 1-800-654-2452 (US). From outside the United States, call 1-314-447-8871. Fax: 1-314-447-8029. E-mail: journalscustomerservice-usa@elsevier.com (for print support) and journalsonlinesupport-usa@elsevier.com (for online support).

Reprints. For copies of 100 or more, of articles in this publication, please contact the Commercial Reprints Department, Elsevier Inc., 360 Park Avenue South, New York, New York 10010-1710. Tel.: 212-633-3874, Fax: 212-633-3820, E-mail: reprints@elsevier.com.

Psychiatric Clinics of North America is covered in *MEDLINE/PubMed (Index Medicus)*, *Current Contents/Social and Behavioral Sciences, Social Science Citation Index, Embase/Excerpta Medica,* and PsycINFO.

Contributors

EDITORS

JOHN M.W. BRADFORD, MD, DPM, FFPsych, DABFP, FRCPC, CM
Institute of Mental Health Research, Brockville Mental Health Centre (BMHC), University of Ottawa, Brockville, Ontario, Canada

A.G. AHMED, MBBS, LLM, MSc, MPsychMed, MRCPsych, FRCPC
Associate Professor, Divisions of Forensic Psychiatry and Addiction and Mental Health, Department of Psychiatry, Institute of Mental Health Research, Brockville Mental Health Centre (BMHC), Associate Chief (Forensic), Royal Ottawa Health Care Group, University of Ottawa, Ottawa, Ontario, Canada

AUTHORS

A.G. AHMED, MBBS, LLM, MSc, MPsychMed, MRCPsych, FRCPC
Associate Professor, Divisions of Forensic Psychiatry and Addiction and Mental Health, Department of Psychiatry, Institute of Mental Health Research, Brockville Mental Health Centre (BMHC), Associate Chief (Forensic), Royal Ottawa Health Care Group, University of Ottawa, Ottawa, Ontario, Canada

ALESSANDRA ALMEIDA ASSUMPÇÃO, BSW
Clinical Psychologist and Social Assistant, Department of Psychiatry, INCT-Medicina Molecular, Programa de Pós-graduação em Medicina Molecular, Universidade Federal de Minas Gerais, Belo Horizonte, Minas Gerais, Brazil

BRAD D. BOOTH, MD, FRCPC, DABPN
Assistant Professor, Department of Psychiatry, University of Ottawa, Ottawa; Psychiatrist, Integrated Forensic Program, Royal Ottawa Mental Health Centre, Royal Ottawa Health Care Group, Ottawa; Director, Sexual Behaviors Unit, St Lawrence Valley Correctional & Treatment Centre, Brockville, Ontario, Canada

DOMINIQUE BOURGET, MD, FRCPC
Associate Professor, Forensic Program, Department of Psychiatry, The Royal Ottawa Hospital, University of Ottawa, Ottawa, Ontario, Canada

JOHN M.W. BRADFORD, MD, DPM, FFPsych, DABFP, FRCPC, CM
Institute of Mental Health Research, Brockville Mental Health Centre (BMHC), University of Ottawa, Brockville, Ontario, Canada

PEER BRIKEN, MD, FECSM
Professor for Sex Research & Forensic Psychiatry, Institute for Sex Research & Forensic Psychiatry, University Medical Centre Hamburg-Eppendorf, University of Hamburg, Hamburg, Germany

MATHIEU DUFOUR, MD, FRCPC
Assistant Professor, Forensic Program, Department of Psychiatry, The Royal Ottawa Hospital, University of Ottawa, Ottawa, Ontario, Canada

PAUL FEDOROFF, MD
Head, Division of Forensic Psychiatry, Director, Sexual Behaviours Clinic, Royal Ottawa Mental Health Centre, University of Ottawa, Ottawa, Canada

FREDERICO DUARTE GARCIA, MD, PhD
Professor, Department of Psychiatry, INCT-Medicina Molecular, Universidade Federal de Minas Gerais, Belo Horizonte, Minas Gerais, Brazil; INSERM U1073, Rouen University Hospital, Rouen University, Rouen, France

HELOISE DELAVENNE GARCIA, MD
Department of Psychiatry, Universidade Federal de Minas Gerais, Belo Horizonte, Minas Gerais, Brazil

DOROTHY M. GRIFFITHS, CM, OOnt, PhD
Co-Director, International Dual Diagnosis Certificate Programme; Professor, Department of Child and Youth Studies, Centre of Applied Disability Studies, Brock University, St Catharines, Ontario, Canada

SANJIV GULATI, MBBS, MRCPsych
Assistant Professor, Department of Psychiatry, University of Ottawa, Ottawa; Psychiatrist, Integrated Forensic Program, Royal Ottawa Mental Health Centre, Royal Ottawa Health Care Group, Ottawa; Director, Assessment & Stabilization Unit, St Lawrence Valley Correctional & Treatment Centre, Brockville, Ontario, Canada

DREW A. KINGSTON, PhD
Royal Ottawa Health Care Group, Ottawa, Ontario, Canada

LIAM ERIC MARSHALL, PhD
Waypoint Centre for Mental Health Care, Penetanguishene, Ontario, Canada

WILLIAM LAMONT MARSHALL, OC, PhD, FRSC
Emeritus Professor, Queen's University, Rockwood Psychological Services, Inverary, Ontario, Canada

MANSFIELD MELA, MBBS, MSc
Associate Professor, Department of Psychiatry, Faculty of Medicine, University of Saskatchewan, Saskatoon, Saskatchewan, Canada

MICHAEL C. SETO, PhD
Director, Forensic Research Unit, uOttawa Institute of Mental Health Research, Royal Ottawa Health Care Group, Ottawa, Ontario, Canada

FLORENCE THIBAUT, MD, PhD
Professor of Psychiatry, Psychiatry and Addictive Disorders, University Hospital Cochin-Tarnier; Faculté de Médecine Paris V Descartes, INSERM U894, Centre des Neurosciences, Paris, France

Contents

Assessment

Michael C. Seto, Drew A. Kingston, and Dominique Bourget

Paraphilias are recurrent, persistent, and intense sexual interests in atypical objects or activities. The most commonly encountered paraphilias in sexological or forensic settings are pedophilia, sexual sadism, exhibitionism, and voyeurism. Paraphilias are often comorbid with other sexual, mood, and personality disorders. Assessment and diagnosis require an integration of multiple sources of clinical information, given the limits and biases of self-report (through clinical interview or questionnaires). Clinicians ideally have access to more objective assessment methods, such as phallometric testing of sexual arousal. The accurate assessment and diagnosis of paraphilias is essential to effective treatment and management.

Treatment

William Lamont Marshall and Liam Eric Marshall

This article describes recent innovations in the psychological treatment of sex offenders. These recent innovations include the incorporation of Andrews and Bonta's *RNR Principles*, Ward's "Good Lives Model," and Miller and Rollnick's *Motivational Interviewing* into a strength-based approach. An example of a strength-based treatment program is described and treatment outcome evaluations are summarized.

Alessandra Almeida Assumpção, Frederico Duarte Garcia,
Heloise Delavenne Garcia, John M.W. Bradford, and Florence Thibaut

The treatment of paraphilias remains a challenge in the mental health field. Combined pharmacologic and psychotherapeutic treatment is associated with better efficacy. The gold standard treatment of severe paraphilias in adult males is antiandrogen treatment with cognitive behavioral therapy. Selective serotonin reuptake inhibitors have been used in mild types of paraphilia and in cases of sexual compulsions and juvenile paraphilias. Antiandrogen treatments seem to be effective in severe paraphilic subjects committing sexual offenses. In particular, gonadotropin-releasing hormone analogs have shown high efficacy working in a similar way to physical castration but being reversible at any time. Treatment recommendations, side effects, and contraindications are discussed.

Sexual offenses with or without aggression attract attention from the popular media and the scientific community. Empirical research suggests a relationship between anger and sexual violence. This article describes the key themes of dysfunctional anger and sexual violence, and how dysfunctional anger relates to sexual fantasies, sexual offending, and sexual recidivism. The implications of the findings for clinical practice and future research are discussed.

Clinicians in sex offender treatment programs always encounter the need to balance the best interests of sex offenders and the safety needs of the community. The protection of the community often takes primacy, resulting in violation of traditional mental health codes of ethics. These ethical dilemmas have generated debates in the academic community. To minimize ethical dilemmas, clinicians in sex offender treatment programs need to acknowledge the conflicts, adhere to safeguards, and thoughtfully address the challenges with profession-specific ethical values and codes. This article reviews ethical principles in relation to conceptualization of sex offenders and their assessment and treatment and research involving sex offenders.

PSYCHIATRIC CLINICS OF NORTH AMERICA

FORTHCOMING ISSUES

September 2014
Obsessive Compulsive Disorder
Wayne Goodman, *Editor*

December 2014
Stress in Health and Disease
Daniel L. Kirsch and
Michel Woodbury, *Editors*

RECENT ISSUES

March 2014
Neuropsychiatry of Traumatic Brain Injury
Ricardo E. Jorge and
David B. Arciniegas, *Editors*

December 2013
Late Life Depression
W. Vaughn McCall, *Editor*

September 2013
Disaster Mental Health: Around the World and Across Time
Craig L. Katz and
Anand Pandya, *Editors*

DOWNLOAD
Free App!

Review Articles
THE CLINICS

NOW AVAILABLE FOR YOUR iPhone and iPad

Psychiatric Clinics of North America

The most current information in Psychiatry from experts in the field

Access online:

www.Psych.TheClinics.com: Personal subscription

www.sciencedirect.com/science/journal/0193953X: Institutional subscription

Access in print:

Individual issues

Subscription of 4 issues annually - one year or multiple year subscription

Take a survey at https://www.surveymonkey.com/s/8R6N9VK

You can be selected for a complimentary one-year personal subscription to the Psychiatric Clinics of North America

Preface

The Natural History of the Paraphilias

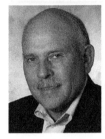 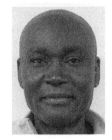

John M.W. Bradford   A.G. Ahmed
Editors

Human sexual behavior is partly the expression of a basic biological drive, the sex drive. Sex drive requires an internal hormonal environment that allows the physiologic expression of sexual behavior. Sexual behaviors principally are there to preserve the species, but in humans, sexual behavior is far more complicated and is associated with our complex social behavior, including emotional expression, emotional bonding, and even to a certain extent, part of recreational activity. Human sexual behavior is linked to and based on neurohormonal development starting in utero and continuing through puberty until the final expression of the behavior occurs in the postpubertal period. Without going into all the neurohormonal factors, androgenization of the male brain occurs at roughly the sixth week of intrauterine life and the male brain is primed differently for males as opposed to females. As androgenization of the brain only occurs in males and deviant sexual behavior is far more common in males at a theoretical level, the androgenization of the brain and the male sexual drive flowing from this neurohormonal process are most likely connected to deviant sexual behavior. Up until puberty, sexual behaviors are experimental and exploratory for the most part. At the time of puberty, with the surge of sexual hormones, sexual drive starts to increase and human sexual behavior becomes activated starting with seeking out a partner for sexual gratification. Individuals are most commonly heterosexual; some are homosexual and some are bisexual. Although this is not fully understood, it does not appear that sexual orientation is learned behavior but is most likely an innate process driven by some complex interactions between androgenization of the brain and neurohormonal changes. In most people sexual behavior then becomes part of their behavioral repertoire as they go forward in life, including establishing relationships and procreation.

A relatively small number of individuals have sexual behavior that deviates significantly from the norm. They go through the same prepubertal period and undergo the same increase in sexual drive as in normal individuals at the time of puberty.

Psychiatr Clin N Am 37 (2014) xi–xv
http://dx.doi.org/10.1016/j.psc.2014.03.010
0193-953X/14/$ – see front matter © 2014 Published by Elsevier Inc.

psych.theclinics.com

The direction of the sexual drive is outside of the normal and is regarded as a sexual deviation, such as the attraction to prepubertal children (pedophilia). This sexual preference manifests as deviant sexual behavior. Even today, we have no real idea as to the prevalence of the various sexual deviations, although some rough estimates have been made for pedophilia. It has always been difficult to estimate prevalence because these behaviors occur in a relatively small number of individuals. Second, as the behavior is deviant from the norm, the behaviors are usually hidden from others and also the behavior may modify with changes in the general structure of society. One of the most recent examples of this is the growth of individuals who seek out child pornography on the Internet. Before the Internet, child pornography was not readily available in print media format. Now, with the development of digital media and the development of the Internet specifically, the access and distribution of child pornography images and videos are much more widespread. One of the questions this raises is whether this is an indication of the prevalence of pedophilia in our current society or is this simply a product of individuals exploring the Internet to view a wide spectrum of digital media depicting sexual acts. Most likely there is a combination of motivations to view pornography on the Internet, including child pornography. Therefore, most likely, not all individuals who view child pornography on the Internet are pedophiles.

Most sexual deviations are regarded as problematic sexual behavior and often involve engaging with nonconsenting individuals, which means it becomes criminal in nature. This means that a number of individuals who have a problem with deviant sexual behavior are also sexual offenders. However, not all sexual offenders have a sexual deviation or paraphilia. In DSM II, sexual deviation was regarded as a personality disorder, but from the evolution of DSM III, it was classified as a psychiatric disorder on Axis I of DSM IIIR[1] and then DSM IV and DSM IVTR.[2] The development of the concept of paraphilia was based on the deviation ("para") and the attraction to the deviation, which is defined by the "philia." In DSM IIIR, paraphilias indicated that unusual or bizarre imagery or acts were necessary for sexual excitement and, in addition, these imagery and acts were persistent and involuntarily repetitive and involved (1) preference for use of nonhuman object; (2) repetitive sexual activity with humans involving real or simulated suffering or humiliation; or (3) repetitive sexual activity with nonconsenting partners. Clearly, this last operational definition involves criminal activity by definition. What was also not clearly defined is that many individuals who have a problem with a sexual deviation also have completely normal sexual behavior. Their sexual preference may be toward the sexual deviation as opposed to a normal sexual outlet but nonetheless both can exist in any given individual.

It also became clear early on that individuals suffering from a paraphilia usually had more than one paraphilia present.[3] In fact, individuals often suffered from two or more paraphilias on a consistent basis and there was a considerable overlap between the different types of paraphilias.[3] This clearly had implications for treatment. The most common form of treatment was psychological and, specifically, behavioral treatment. This type of approach required a specific treatment program for each paraphilia administered one at a time. Psychological treatment involving this technique therefore was more complicated and more prolonged. Pharmacologic treatment started to develop with the principal aim of treatment being the suppression of sexual drive. Sexual drive includes sexual fantasies and urges as well as behavior and all of these elements were suppressed with the pharmacologic intervention. Furthermore, the suppression of deviant sexual fantasies urges and behavior was across the board for any paraphilias that were present in any given individual. The expression of paraphilias also has some cultural dimensions. Frotteurism, inappropriate touching of the nonconsenting female, is not acceptable in North American culture, whereas in some European cultures it may be acceptable.

DSM IV principally maintained the definitions of the paraphilias in DSM III and DSM IIIR.[1,2] However, with the development of DSM V, there has been a considerable shift from DSM IV.[4] There is now differentiation between a paraphilia and a paraphilic disorder. Paraphilia denotes any intense and persistent sexual interest other than sexual interest in genital stimulation or preparatory fondling between phenotypically the normal physically mature, consenting partners.[4] Paraphilic disorder is a paraphilia that is causing distress or impairment to the individual or a paraphilia whose satisfaction has entailed personal harm, or risk of harm, to others.[4] The paraphilic disorders consist of voyeuristic disorder; exhibitionistic disorder; frotteuristic disorder; sexual masochism disorder; sexual sadism disorder; pedophilic disorder; fetishistic disorder; and transvestic disorder.[4] There are other paraphilic disorders that are not specifically named.[4] The first group of disorders is based on anomalous activity preferences.[4] These are further divided into courtship disorders (voyeuristic disorder, exhibitionistic disorder, and frotteuristic disorder) and algolagnic disorders (sexual masochism disorder and sexual sadism disorder). The second group of disorders is based on anomalous target preferences (pedophilic disorder, fetishistic disorder, and transvestic disorder).[4] The actual diagnostic criteria for paraphilic disorders remained mostly the same. The qualitative nature of the paraphilia (criterion A) means that recurrent and intense sexual arousal must be present for at least six months. Criterion B requires that the individual has acted on the sexual urges with a nonconsenting person, or the sexual urges or fantasies cause clinically significant distress or impairment in social, occupational, or other important areas of functioning. In summary, deviant arousal patterns are accompanied by clinically significant distress or impairment. To meet the criteria for a paraphilic disorder, the individual must meet both criterion A and criterion B.

Although the etiology of the paraphilias is not understood, the possibility of neurohormonal difficulties and a genetic predisposition has been explored.[5,6] At this time, the actual cause of the paraphilias is unknown.[5,7]

More recently, a task force of the World Federation of Societies of Biological Psychiatry completed an evidence-based review of the complete literature related to the biological treatment of the paraphilias.[8] This task force also developed an algorithm for treatment based on evidence-based studies, which should assist in the systematic treatment of the paraphilias in the future.[8]

Considerable research has been related to sexual offender recidivism and predicting sexual offender recidivism in different individuals suffering from paraphilic disorders.[9-16] The evaluation of individuals with paraphilias using sexual preference techniques has been important from a diagnostic point of view but also from the point of view predicting recidivism.[14,15,17] This publication reviews many aspects of the paraphilias from both an assessment and a treatment point of view and should help the general psychiatric practitioner to understand and treat paraphilias and paraphilic disorders better.

John M.W. Bradford, MD, DPM, FFPsych, DABFP, FRCPC, CM
Institute of Mental Health Research
University of Ottawa
Brockville Mental Health Centre (BMHC)
1804 Highway 2 East
Brockville, Ontario, K6V 5W7, Canada

A.G. Ahmed, MBBS, LLM, MSc, MPsychMed, MRCPsych, FRCPC
Institute of Mental Health Research
University of Ottawa
Brockville Mental Health Centre (BMHC)
1804 Highway 2 East
Brockville, Ontario, K6V 5W7, Canada

E-mail addresses:
john.Bradford@theroyal.ca (J.M.W. Bradford)
ag.ahmed@theroyal.ca (A.G. Ahmed)

REFERENCES

1. American Psychiatric Association. Diagnostic and statistical manual of mental disorders. 3rd edition. Washington, DC: American Psychiatric Association; 1980.
2. American Psychiatric Association. Diagnostic and statistical manual of mental disorders. 4th edition. Washington, DC: American Psychiatric Association; 1994.
3. Bradford JM, Boulet J, Pawlak A. The paraphilias: a multiplicity of deviant behaviours. Can J Psychiatry 1992;37(2):104–8.
4. American Psychiatric Association. Diagnostic and statistical manual of mental disorders. 5th edition. Washington, DC: American Psychiatric Association; 2013.
5. Labelle A, Bourget D, Bradford JM, et al. Familial paraphilia: a pilot study with the construction of genograms. ISRN Psychiatry 2012;2012:692813.
6. Kingston DA, Seto MC, Ahmed AG, et al. The role of central and peripheral hormones in sexual and violent recidivism in sex offenders. J Am Acad Psychiatry Law 2012;40(4):476–85.
7. Bradford JM. The neurobiology, neuropharmacology, and pharmacological treatment of the paraphilias and compulsive sexual behaviour. Can J Psychiatry 2001;46(1):26–34.
8. Thibaut F, De La Barra F, Gordon H, et al. The World Federation of Societies of Biological Psychiatry (WFSBP) guidelines for the biological treatment of paraphilias. World J Biol Psychiatry 2010;11(4):604–55.
9. Kingston DA, Seto MC, Ahmed AG, et al. Comparing indicators of sexual sadism as predictors of recidivism among adult male sexual offenders. J Consult Clin Psychol 2010;78(4):574–84.
10. Kingston DA, Yates PM, Firestone P, et al. Pornography use and sexual aggression: the impact of frequency and type of pornography use on recidivism among sexual offenders. Aggress Behav 2008;34(4):341–51.
11. Nunes KL, Hanson RK, Firestone P, et al. Denial predicts recidivism for some sexual offenders. Sex Abuse 2007;19(2):91–105.
12. Nunes KL, Firestone P, Wexler AF, et al. Incarceration and recidivism among sexual offenders. Law Hum Behav 2007;31(3):305–18.
13. Kingston DA, Firestone P, Moulden HM, et al. The utility of the diagnosis of pedophilia: a comparison of various classification procedures. Arch Sex Behav 2007;36(3):423–36.
14. Firestone P, Kingston DA, Wexler A, et al. Long-term follow-up of exhibitionists: psychological, phallometric, and offense characteristics. J Am Acad Psychiatry Law 2006;34(3):349–59.
15. Greenberg DM, Firestone P, Nunes KL, et al. Biological fathers and stepfathers who molest their daughters: psychological, phallometric, and criminal features. Sex Abuse 2005;17(1):39–46.

16. Firestone P, Nunes KL, Moulden H, et al. Hostility and recidivism in sexual offenders. Arch Sex Behav 2005;34(3):277–83.
17. Firestone P, Dixon KL, Nunes KL, et al. A comparison of incest offenders based on victim age. J Am Acad Psychiatry Law 2005;33(2):223–32.

Assessment of the Paraphilias

Michael C. Seto, PhD*, Drew A. Kingston, PhD, Dominique Bourget, MD

KEYWORDS

- Paraphilias • Pedophilia • Sexual sadism • Assessment • Diagnosis

KEY POINTS

- Paraphilias are recurrent, persistent, and intense sexual interests in atypical objects or activities.
- Although they are most often seen in forensic or sexological settings, paraphilias can be encountered in general psychiatric settings as well.
- Paraphilias have significant comorbidity, both with other paraphilias and with mood disorders in particular.
- Assessment and diagnosis require integration of multiple sources of information given the limits and biases of self-report alone.
- Effective management of paraphilias requires ongoing monitoring because there is no evidence that the condition can be cured.

INTRODUCTION
Definition

Paraphilias are defined in the latest version of the Diagnostic and Statistical Manual of Mental Disorders (DSM) as recurrent and intense sexual arousal to atypical objects or activities, as manifested in sexual fantasies, urges, or behavior over at least a 6-month period.[1,2] In the DSM, Fifth Edition (DSM-5), paraphilias are distinct from paraphilic disorders; the latter term denotes a paraphilia that is accompanied by distress or impairment in functioning. Paraphilias are necessary but not sufficient for determining the presence of a paraphilic disorder.[1]

Eight paraphilias are specifically listed in the DSM-5: pedophilia (prepubescent children), exhibitionism (exposing the genitals to an unsuspecting stranger), voyeurism (spying on unsuspecting strangers in normally private activities), sexual sadism (inflicting humiliation, bondage, or suffering), sexual masochism (experiencing humiliation, bondage, or suffering); frotteurism (touching/rubbing against an unconsenting

Disclosures: None.
Royal Ottawa Health Care Group, uOttawa Institute of Mental Health Research, 1145 Carling Avenue, Ottawa, Ontario K1Z 7K4, Canada
* Corresponding author. Integrated Forensic Program, Royal Ottawa Health Care Group, 1804 Highway 2 East, Brockville, Ontario K6V 5W7, Canada.
E-mail address: michael.seto@theroyal.ca

Psychiatr Clin N Am 37 (2014) 149–161
http://dx.doi.org/10.1016/j.psc.2014.03.001
0193-953X/14/$ – see front matter © 2014 Elsevier Inc. All rights reserved.

Abbreviations	
BSHI	Bradford Sexual History Inventory
CPA	Cyproterone acetate
DSM	Diagnostic and Statistical Manual of Mental Disorders
LA	Leuprolide acetate
MIDSA	Multidimensional Inventory of Development, Sex, and Aggression
MPA	Medroxyprogesterone acetate
MSI	Multiphasic Sex Inventory
OCD	Obsessive-compulsive disorder
PPG	Phallometry or penile plethysmography
SHQ-R	Clarke Sex History Questionnaire for Males–Revised
SSPI	Screening Scale for Pedophilic Interests

person), fetishism (nongenital body parts or nonliving objects), and transvestism (cross-dressing). Many other paraphilias have been described in clinical case studies. In DSM-5, these other paraphilias are diagnosed as other specified paraphilia if the atypical focus is known, or as unspecified paraphilia if there are clear symptoms that warrant the diagnosis of a paraphilic disorder but the clinician either cannot or does not want to specify the paraphilic focus. Similar descriptions of paraphilias are included in the tenth version of the International Classification of Diseases, which is more commonly used outside Canada and the United States.[3,4]

Nature of the Problem

Paraphilic disorders are most commonly seen in forensic and correctional settings, when paraphilic behaviors are illegal if acted on, such as accessing child pornography or having sexual contact with a child.[5,6] Other paraphilias that are commonly seen in forensic and correctional settings include exhibitionism, voyeurism, and sexual sadism. We have also seen fetishists when their sexual interests lead them to engage in criminal behavior; for example, when an underwear fetishist breaks into women's residences in order to steal underwear. Paraphilias are also often seen in sexological settings, especially when they lead to impairment in sexual or relationship functioning. For example, sexual masochism might be seen when someone is in a long-term, committed relationship with someone who does not tolerate the interest or will not engage in masochistic activities. Because paraphilias can affect sexual and relationship functioning and because they are highly comorbid with mood problems, individuals with paraphilias experiencing these consequences might be seen in any general psychiatric setting. An unknown proportion of paraphilic individuals do not seek consultation.

Prevalence

The prevalence of paraphilias is not known, although there are some relevant studies. Långström and Seto[7] analyzed data from 2450 randomly selected men and women from 18 to 60 years of age in Sweden. Seventy-six respondents (3.1%) reported at least one incident of being sexually aroused by exposing their genitals to a stranger, and 191 (7.7%) respondents reported at least one incident of being sexually aroused by spying on others having sex. Beier and colleagues[8] conducted an anonymous survey of 373 men, and 4% admitted having sexual contact with a child, 9% admitting having sexual fantasies about children, and 6% admitted masturbating to fantasies about children. Richters and colleagues[9] conducted a large telephone survey in which 2% of male respondents and 1.4% of female respondents reported engaging in sadistic or masochistic activities in the past 12 months.

These studies provide upper-limit bounds for prevalence because the surveys did not include items about recurrence, intensity, or persistence. Seto[6] reviewed the pedophilia literature and inferred an upper-limit prevalence of pedophilia in community settings ranging from 1% to 3% in men. The prevalence of paraphilic disorder is necessarily lower than the prevalence of paraphilias, because some individuals do not experience distress or impairment as a result of their interest.

Symptoms/Criteria

Paraphilic disorders have commonalities across criteria. The first overlap is that there is recurrent and intense sexual arousal from the paraphilic focus for at least 6 months, and the second common criterion is that the person engages in paraphilic behavior involving a nonconsenting person or the accompanying sexual fantasies or urges cause clinically significant distress or impairment in functioning.

Paraphilic disorder diagnoses are usually reserved for adults because of a reluctance to apply a stigmatizing label to adolescents. There is also a widely held notion that adolescence is a period of fluidity in sexual development, and thus the persistence aspect of paraphilias and paraphilic disorders is not clearly established. Of the 8 specified paraphilic disorders, 2 have age criteria: voyeuristic disorder is not to be diagnosed before the age of 18 years; and pedophilic disorder is not to be diagnosed before the age of 16 years, and only if there is at least a 5-year age difference between the individual and the child.

CLINICAL FINDINGS

Assessment and diagnosis of paraphilias requires a comprehensive, multimodal examination, including a mental status examination to screen for any co-occurring psychiatric conditions; review of sexual history via interview and questionnaires; a sex hormone profile; and ideally psychophysiologic testing of sexual arousal patterns (**Table 1**). Collateral information from current or former sexual partners and from files is invaluable because of the limits of self-report, especially if there are legal or other consequences. However, self-report is still essential because it can provide firsthand information about sexual thoughts, fantasies, and urges. Honest self-report is more likely when evaluators are warm, nonjudgmental, and able to ask sexuality questions sensitively.

Physical Examination

A sex hormone profile screens for abnormal hormone levels and establishes a baseline level for any pharmacologic treatment. The profile consists of free and total testosterone, follicle-stimulating hormone, luteinizing hormone, estradiol, prolactin, and progesterone.[15,16] Some of these hormones have shown usefulness in predicting recidivism among sexual offenders.[17,18]

Pharmacologic intervention to reduce sexual drive and thus inhibit sexual behavior is warranted for high-risk paraphilic sex offenders. In advance of treatment of paraphilia, screening tests can minimize possible medical complications before using antiandrogens, including cyproterone acetate (CPA) and medroxyprogesterone acetate (MPA), and the luteinizing hormone–releasing hormone agonist leuprolide acetate (LA). For CPA and MPA, contraindications include thromboembolic disorders and active pituitary disorders.[19] Both CPA and MPA can cause liver damage and are contraindicated in individuals with abnormal liver function.[20,21] Contraindications for LA include osteoporosis and active pituitary disorders.[19]

Table 1
Self-report sexual interest measures

Test (Source)	Description	Domains Included in the Measure
BSHI[10]	The BSHI is a comprehensive measure that consists of 81 items that have been grouped into 9 categories. This measure has been used in several studies with sexual offenders to assess various types of paraphilias and other related constructs	There are no predefined categories. Each section pertains to a variety of sexual interests and experiences across various developmental stages
MIDSA[11]	The MIDSA is a computerized inventory that has been used with both adult and juvenile sexual offenders. The MIDSA is the most comprehensive computerized assessment inventory available and includes 53 subscales. The MIDSA covers 16 domains, such as criminal behavior, deviant sexual interests and behaviors, and personality traits (eg, psychopathy). The measure has shown excellent psychometric properties, which have been reported in several empirical studies	Criminal and other antisocial behavior and values; developmental history and family background; deviant sexual interests and arousal; education and employment histories; peer and romantic relationship history; relevant personality traits; sexual history; substance use; use of sexually arousing materials; history of aggression or violence; history of sexually abusive behavior; level of cognitive functioning and other responsivity factors; level of self-disclosure and accountability; official and unreported history of sexual and nonsexual crimes; insight into offense precursors and risk; medical and mental health history
MSI[12]	The MSI is a 300-item measure used to assess a full range of sexual preferences and sexual behaviors. Kalichman et al[13] reported good internal consistency, construct validity, and discriminant validity. The MSI has been updated and expanded (MSI-II) and includes 560 true/false questions. In addition to the 10 core scales of the MSI listed in the adjacent column, the revised tool includes additional reliability/validity, psychosexual, behavioral, and accountability measures. See www.nicholsandmolinder.com for psychometric properties on the newly revised tool	1. Child molestation 2. Rape 3. Exhibitionism 4. Fetishism 5. Voyeurism 6. Bondage/discipline 7. Sadomasochism 8. Sexual dysfunction 9. Sex knowledge 10. Treatment attitudes
SHQ-R[14]	The SHQ-R is a comprehensive self-report measure that assesses a wide range of sexual interests and behaviors. The measure includes 508 items in a multiple-choice response format that have been reduced, via factor analyses, to 23 scales	Childhood and adolescent sexual experiences and sexual abuse; sexual dysfunction; female adult frequency; female pubescent frequency; female child frequency; male adult frequency; male pubescent frequency; male child frequency; child identification; fantasy activities with women; fantasy activities with men; exposure to pornography; transvestism; fetishism; feminine gender identity; voyeurism; exhibitionism frequency; exhibiting behavior; obscene phone calls; frotteurism; sexual aggression; lie; infrequency

Abbreviations: BSHI, Bradford Sexual History Inventory; MIDSA, The Multidimensional Inventory of Development, Sex, and Aggression; MSI, The Multiphasic Sex Inventory; SHQ-R, Clarke Sex History Questionnaire for Males Revised

Psychophysiologic Methods

Phallometry

Phallometry, or penile plethysmography (PPG), involves the measurement of changes in penile circumference or volume in response to stimuli that vary on the particular dimension of interest (eg, age, level of violence). Multiple studies show that phallometrically assessed sexual arousal to children is useful in the assessment of pedophilia and hebephilia.[5,22,23] Relative sexual arousal to children distinguishes sex offenders with child victims from other men, including sex offenders with adult victims, nonsex offenders, and nonoffending controls. Moreover, relative sexual arousal to children is one of the most robust predictors of sexual recidivism among sex offenders.[24]

There also are multiple studies showing that rapists can be distinguished from other men in their relative response to depictions of sexual coercion and violence.[25] A controversy is the extent to which this represents a specific paraphilia, which Lalumiere and colleagues[25] described as biastophilia (a preference for coercive sex), or is a variant or manifestation of sexual sadism. In 2 recent studies, Seto and colleagues[26,27] and Harris and colleagues[28,29] suggested that rapists are more sexually aroused by cues of coercion than by physical violence or suffering, whereas the opposite was true for self-identified sexual sadists.

Most phallometric research has focused on pedophilia, biastophilia, and sexual sadism, because child molesters and rapists are the most common types of sex offenders seen clinically. Marshall and Fernandez[30] reviewed 10 phallometric studies of exhibitionists and found that only 1 revealed evidence of a preference for genital exposing. However, other studies have revealed group differences between male exhibitionists and other men.[31] There are also individual studies supporting the usefulness of phallometric testing for fetishism[32] and sexual masochism.[33]

Viewing time

Phallometric testing is effective but it has been criticized because it is expensive, assessees dislike the procedure, and it can be difficult to gain access. A Safer Society survey of treatment providers found that a minority of sex offender treatment programs used phallometric testing, ranging from 28% of the 330 community programs to 36% of the 85 residential programs serving adult men.[34] As a result, there has been interest in developing alternative methods that are still objective and difficult to fake. An increasingly common method involves the presentation of pictures of semi-clothed children, adolescents, or adults (swimsuits) and the covert recording of relative viewing time.[35–39] In conjunction with responses to a computer-administered questionnaire, sex offenders with child victims are distinguished from other men.[35,40] Viewing time is more common than phallometry in community programs, whereas phallometry is more common in residential programs.[34] We are not aware of viewing time paradigms that can assess paraphilias other than pedophilia or hebephilia. There is much less evidence on the predictive validity of viewing time measures. A recent study suggested that viewing time scores significantly predict sexual recidivism.[41,42]

Rating Scales

Self-report of sexual interests

Assessees should be questioned about their sexual thoughts, interests, and behaviors via clinical interview. Interviews can be informative, particularly when a respondent admits to atypical sexual interests and behaviors. Some individuals may be reluctant to disclose personal sexual information, particularly if the behaviors are atypical and if the answers may result in negative consequences. One way to reduce the reluctance of individuals to disclose their sexual interests is to administer self-report question-naires. There are several inventories designed to assess sexual interest, a few of which are described next.

The Multidimensional Inventory of Development, Sex, and Aggression The Multidimensional Inventory of Development, Sex, and Aggression (MIDSA) is a computerized inventory for use with adults with sexual behavior problems.[11,43] The MIDSA has 53 subscales that were developed using factor analysis and rational scale construction. The MIDSA includes an exhaustive list of questions pertaining to specific life experiences, subjective emotional states, sexual fantasies, attitudes, behavioral proclivities, and cognitions. The MIDSA has undergone extensive validation since its initial version, the Multidimensional Assessment of Sexual Aggression,[44] and recent studies have supported the validity of the measure (see Refs.[11,43,45–50]). Among adult sexual offenders, the internal consistency of all scales across the 14 domains exceeded 0.65 and most scales produced coefficients between 0.85 and 0.95. Studies have similarly shown adequate test-retest reliability with coefficients exceeding 0.75 across all scales. The measure has also shown excellent concurrent validity with other scales measuring similar constructs.[11,45]

The Multiphasic Sex Inventory The Multiphasic Sex Inventory (MSI) is a 300-item, true/false instrument used widely with sexual offenders.[12] The MSI generates 20 scale scores that measure interest in a variety of paraphilias, including pedophilia, coercive sex, exhibitionism, fetishism, and sadomasochism. The MSI has shown good psychometric properties[13] and the scales are able to differentiate types of sexual offenders.[12] Craig and colleagues[51] reported that certain subscales (Sexual Deviance Factor, Sexual Obsessions, Sexual/Social Desirability, and Sexual Dysfunction) were able to predict recidivism. The MSI has been updated (MSI-II) to include 560 true/false questions.[52] However, there is limited research available on the validity of the revised measure, although the test developers provide some psychometric data (see www. nicholsandmolinder.com).

Clarke Sex History Questionnaire The Clarke Sex History Questionnaire for Males–Revised (SHQ-R) is a 508-item measure of sexual and personal history.[14] Items are in a multiple-choice format and have been grouped into 23 scales that pertain to a variety of domains, including childhood and adolescent experiences, sexual dysfunction, adult age/gender sexual outlets, fantasy and pornography, transvestism, fetishism, female gender identity disorder, and courtship disorder. Several studies have reported the instrument to be psychometrically sound.[14,53]

Bradford Sexual History Inventory The Bradford Sexual History Inventory (BSHI) consists of 81 items grouped into 9 categories.[10] The psychometric properties have not been published but it has been used clinically for some time, and information obtained from the BSHI has been reported in several studies with sexual offenders.[17,54–57]

Clinician ratings of sexual victim history
Screening Scale for Pedophilic Interests The Screening Scale for Pedophilic Interests (SSPI) is based on sexual child victim characteristics and is moderately associated with PPG and other measures of sexual interest in children.[58–62] The SSPI was initially developed using a sample of 1113 sexual offenders against children. Four victim characteristics were selected because they were easily coded and independently contributed to the prediction of phallometrically assessed sexual arousal to children: (1) any boy victims; (2) more than one child victim; (3) having a victim aged 11 years or younger; and (4) having an unrelated child victim.

These 4 variables are scored as present or absent, using all available information about sexual offenses, but drawing primarily from files. Each item has a score of 0 or 1, except for boy victims, which has a score of 0 or 2. Thus, sex offenders with child victims can have an SSPI score ranging from 0 to 5. An example of someone with a score of 0 is an incest offender with a single girl victim aged 13 years; an example of someone with a score of 5 is an offender with multiple child victims, at least one of them a boy, unrelated, and aged 11 years or younger. Offenders with a score of 5 are approximately 5 times more likely to be pedophilic than offenders with a score of 0. Recent studies have replicated Seto and Lalumière's[58] initial findings and have shown that SSPI scores can predict new sexual offenses committed by sexual offenders against children (eg, Refs.[62], Helmus L, O'Ciardha C, Seto MC. The Screening Scale for Pedophilic Interests (SSPI): Construct, predictive, and incremental validity. 2013. Submitted for publication).

DIAGNOSTIC DILEMMAS
Process of Elimination

It is important to distinguish between reported fantasies and urges inherent to paraphilias and obsessional sexual thoughts associated with obsessive-compulsive disorder (OCD). Unacceptable or taboo thoughts, including sexual or aggressive obsessions, are recognized as a distinct symptom profile in OCD. These obsessional thoughts are often accompanied by compulsions.[63–65] Glazier and colleagues[66] found that mental health professionals commonly misidentified taboo obsessional thoughts, particularly those of a sexual nature, and noted that limited awareness of OCD presentations could explain the misidentifications. Brakoulias and colleagues[67] suggested that taboo thoughts might be characterized by higher levels of hostility and of past (nonalcohol) substance dependence.

Inter-rater Reliability

Research on the DSM-IV Text Revision (DSM-IV-TR) criteria for pedophilia (unchanged in DSM-5) indicates moderate inter-rater reliability, possibly affected by the evaluators being involved with opposing sides in high-stakes and adversarial legal proceedings.[68] The inter-rater reliabilities for sexual sadism and exhibitionism were poorer in this study. Other data also suggest moderate reliability at best.[69] In contrast, Doren and Elwood[70] found good inter-rater reliability for the sexual sadism diagnosis in using detailed case descriptions of 12 sex offenders in a sample of 34 evaluators, and some recent unpublished data suggest adequate, if not excellent, inter-rater reliability.[71,72] Many clinicians and researchers have called for more inter-rater reliability studies of DSM paraphilia criteria.

Comorbidities

Paraphilias tend to co-occur, such that someone with a paraphilia is more likely to engage in other paraphilic behavior than someone who is randomly drawn from the general population. For example, 2 studies have shown that some pedophiles also engage in exhibitionistic (12%–13%) or voyeuristic (11%–36%) behavior.[73,74] Freund and colleagues[75] observed that certain paraphilias (voyeurism, exhibitionism, and frotteurism) are more likely to co-occur with each other than with other paraphilias. For example, two-thirds of the 144 frotteurs in their clinical sample showed exhibitionistic or voyeuristic behavior. Freund[76] suggested a courtship disorder model to explain why these paraphilias "hang together." In addition, some community surveys also suggest overlap in paraphilic behavior; Långström and Seto[77] found higher co-occurrence of exhibitionistic and voyeuristic behavior than expected by chance. This evidence of co-occurrence of paraphilic behavior suggests common causal factors across para-philias. One commonality might be hypersexuality, because hypersexuality was asso-ciated with exhibitionistic, voyeurism, and other paraphilic behavior by Långström and Hanson.[78]

There is also evidence that paraphilias are often comorbid with other psychiatric conditions. For example, Kafka and Hennen[79] examined 88 paraphilic individuals (60 had committed sexual offenses) and found high comorbidity for any mood disorder (72%), any anxiety disorder (39%), and attention-deficit/hyperactivity disorder (ADHD) (42%). In sexual offenders in forensic psychiatric settings, psychiatric disorders are prevalent, including personality disorders.[80–85] McElroy and colleagues[84] reported that 28 of the 36 sexual offenders (78%) in their sample had 3 or more comorbid axis I disorders: disorders of mood, anxiety and eating were seen more often in para-philic versus nonparaphilic sexual offenders. Substance use disorders were also common.

Leue and colleagues[82] noted that anxiety, mood, and substance abuse disorders were common in 55 sexual offenders, 30 of whom were classified as having a para-philia disorder and 25 of whom were classified as having an impulse control disorder (without paraphilia). Social phobia was more prevalent among paraphilic offenders, whereas major depression occurred most often in the impulse control–disordered group. In a recent review, Kafka[86] suggested that substance use disorder and mood disorders were highly prevalent among adult male paraphilic offenders. In adolescent sexual offenders, posttraumatic stress disorder, conduct disorder, and ADHD and other neurodevelopmental disorders (eg, Asperger disorder and fetal alcohol spectrum disorder) were reported as common.

Case Studies

Case 1

JK was a 27-year-old married man, father of a 3-year-old daughter, who presented to an outpatient sexology clinic in acute distress after his wife threatened separation. The couple had been married for 5 years. JK revealed that he obtained sexual arousal from soiled diapers. His wife had agreed to participate in role playing in which he pretended to be a child and defecated in a diaper. At this juncture, she was no longer willing to be involved in this activity. She further expressed concerns because he had started to use their daughter's diapers as an arousing stimulus for his masturbatory activity. He had on occasions hired prostitutes willing to assist him in fulfilling his fantasies. However, he had become fearful for his reputation as a small business owner. Over the last 7 years, JK had attended several doctors' offices and he had consulted 3 different psychologists for psychotherapy and several treatment modalities, all of which failed to produce any result. Although he expressed his desire to modify his behavior, his motivation to seek treatment was solely external. After his wife decided to remain in the relationship for the welfare of their daughter, he chose not to pursue any follow-up treatment.

Case 2

JS was a 27-year-old, unmarried man attending a sex offender treatment program as part of his criminal sentence for sexually offending against a boy. File information indi-cated he gave alcohol to a 13-year-old boy after befriending the boy's mother, and performed fellatio on the boy after the boy fell asleep. The boy woke up while this was happening and ran out of the apartment. On entering treatment, JS denied he had committed the sexual offense, claiming the conviction was a result of a misunderstanding. He was assessed phallometrically and was found to have strong sexual arousal to depictions of young boys and little sexual arousal to adult men or women. During his treatment, JS admitted to previously undetected sexual interactions with dozens of boys, beginning in his own childhood after he was sexually abused by older boys. JS was diagnosed with pedophilia and underwent cognitive behavioral treatment of this condition, and for his sexual offending.

SUMMARY

Paraphilias are most likely to be encountered in forensic or sexological settings, but they can be seen in any general psychiatric setting. Assessment and diagnosis require careful attention to multiple sources of information, including interview, questionnaire, a medical examination, and psychophysiologic testing. Given the challenges in interrater agreement, detailed notes about the sources of information and how they inform the diagnosis are important.

REFERENCES

1. American Psychiatric Association. Diagnostic and statistical manual of mental disorders. 5th edition. Washington, DC: American Psychiatric Association; 2013.
2. Babchishin KM, Nunes KL, Kessous N. A multimodal examination of sexual interest in children: a comparison of sex offenders and non-sex offenders. Sex Abuse 2013. http://dx.doi.org/10.1177/1079063213492343. Advance online publication.
3. World Health Organization. International statistical classification of diseases and related health problems (10th rev.). 2010. Available at: http://apps.who.int/classifications/icd10/browse/2010/en. Accessed March 24, 2014.
4. Worling JR. Assessing sexual arousal with adolescent males who have offended sexually: self-report and unobtrusively measured viewing time. Sex Abuse 2006; 18:383–400. http://dx.doi.org/10.1007/s11194-006-9024-1.
5. Seto MC. Pedophilia and sexual offending against children: theory, assessment, and intervention. Washington, DC: American Psychological Association; 2008.
6. Seto MC. Internet sex offenders. Washington, DC: American Psychological Association; 2013.
7. Seto MC, Cantor JM, Blanchard R. Child pornography offenses are a valid diagnostic indicator of pedophilia. J Abnorm Psychol 2006;115:610–5.
8. Beier KM, Neutze J, Mundt IA, et al. Encouraging self-identified pedophiles and hebephiles to seek professional help: first results of the Prevention Project Dunkelfeld (PPD). Child Abuse Negl 2009;33:545–9.
9. Richters J, De Visser RO, Rissel CE, et al. Demographic and psychosocial features of participants in bondage and discipline, "sadomasochism" or dominance and submission (BDSM): data from a national survey. J Sex Med 2008; 5:1660–8.
10. Bradford JMW, Pawlak A, Boulet JR, et al. Bradford Sexual History Inventory (BSHI). Ottawa, Ontario, Canada: Royal Ottawa Hospital; 2002. Unpublished inventory.
11. Multidimensional Inventory of Development, Sex, and Aggression (MIDSA). MIDSA clinical manual. Bend (OR): Augur Enterprises; 2011. Available at: http://www.midsa.us.
12. Nichols H, Molinder I. Manual for the multiphasic sex inventory. Tacoma (WA): Crime and Victim Psychology Specialists; 1984.

13. Kalichman SC, Henderson MC, Shealy LS, et al. Psychometric properties of the Multiphasic Sex Inventory in assessing sex offenders. Crim Justice Behav 1992; 19:384–96.

14. Langevin R, Paitich D. Clarke sex history questionnaire for males-revised (SHQ-R). North Tonawanda (NY): Multi-Health Systems; 2002.

15. Bourget D, Bradford JM. Evidential basis for the assessment and treatment of sex offenders. Brief Treat Crisis Interv 2008;8:130–46.

16. Blanchard R, Klassen P, Dickey R, et al. Sensitivity and specificity of the phallometric test for pedophilia in nonadmitting sex offenders. Psychol Assess 2001; 13:118–26.

17. Kingston DA, Seto MC, Ahmed AG, et al. Central and peripheral hormones in sexual and violent recidivism in sexual offenders. J Am Acad Psychiatry Law 2012;40:476–85.

18. Studer LH, Aylwin AS, Reddon JR. Testosterone, sexual offense recidivism, and treatment effect among adult male sex offenders. Sex Abuse 2005;17:171–81.

19. Guay DR. Drug treatment of paraphilic and nonparaphilic sexual disorders. Clin Ther 2009;31:1–31.

20. Reilly DR, Delva NJ, Hudson RW. Protocols for the use of cyproterone, medroxyprogesterone, and leuprolide in the treatment of paraphilia. Can J Psychiatry 2000;45:559–63.

21. Rice ME, Harris GT, Lang C, et al. Adolescents who have sexually offended: is phallometry valid? Sex Abuse 2012;24:133–52.

22. Seto MC. Pedophilia. Annu Rev Clin Psychol 2009;5:391–407. http://dx.doi.org/10.1146/annurev.clinpsy.032408.153618.

23. Seto MC. Child pornography use and internet solicitation in the diagnosis of pedophilia. Arch Sex Behav 2010;39:591–3. http://dx.doi.org/10.1007/s10508-010-9603-6.

24. Hanson RK, Morton-Bourgon KE. The characteristics of persistent sexual offenders: a meta-analysis of recidivism studies. J Consult Clin Psychol 2005; 73:1154–63.

25. Lalumiere ML, Harris GT, Quinsey VL, et al. The causes of rape: understanding individual differences in male propensity for sexual aggression. Washington, DC: American Psychological Association; 2005.

26. Seto MC, Lalumière ML, Harris GT, et al. The sexual responses of sexual sadists. J Abnorm Psychol 2012;121:739–53.

27. Seto MC, Murphy WD, Page J, et al. Detecting anomalous sexual interests in juvenile sex offenders. Ann N Y Acad Sci 2003;989:118–30. http://dx.doi.org/10.1111/j.1749-6632.2003.tb07298.x.

28. Harris GT, Lalumière ML, Seto MC, et al. The sexual arousal of rapists to rape stories: the contributions of sex, nonconsent, and injury. Arch Sex Behav 2012.

29. Harris GT, Rice ME. The science in phallometric testing of male sexual interest. Curr Dir Psychol Sci 1996;5:156–60.

30. Marshall WL, Fernandez YM. Sexual preferences: are they useful in the assessment and treatment of sexual offenders? Aggress Violent Behav 2003;8:131–43.

31. Marshall WL, Payne K, Barbaree HE, et al. Exhibitionists: sexual preferences for exposing. Behav Res Ther 1991;29:37–40.

32. Freund K, Seto MC, Kuban M. Two types of fetishism. Behav Res Ther 1996;34:687–94.

33. Chivers ML, Roy C, Grimbos T, et al. Specificity of sexual arousal for sexual activities in men and women with conventional and masochistic sexual interests [online first]. Arch Sex Behav 2013. [Epub ahead of print].

34. McGrath R, Cumming G, Burchard B, et al. Current practices and emerging trends in sexual abuser management: the Safer Society 2009 North American survey. Brandon (VT): Safer Society; 2010.

35. Abel GG, Huffman J, Warberg B, et al. Visual reaction time and plethysmography as measures of sexual interest in child molesters. Sex Abuse 1998;10: 81–95. http://dx.doi.org/10.1023/A:1022063214826.

36. Harris GT, Rice ME, Quinsey VL, et al. Viewing time as a measure of sexual interest among child molesters and normal heterosexual men. Behav Res Ther 1996;34:389–94.

37. Harris GT, Rice ME, Quinsey VL, et al. Maximizing the discriminant validity of phallometric assessment. Psychol Assess 1992;4:502–11.

38. Hill A, Habermann N, Berner W, et al. Psychiatric disorders in single and multiple sexual murderers. Psychopathology 2006;40:22–8.

39. Holt SE, Meloy JR, Strack S. Sadism and psychopathy in violent and sexually violent offenders. J Am Acad Psychiatry Law 1999;27:23–32.

40. Glasgow DV. Affinity: the development of a self-report assessment of paedophile sexual interest incorporating a viewing time measure. In: Thornton D, Laws DR, editors. Cognitive approaches to the assessment of sexual interest in sexual offenders. Chichester (United Kingdom): Wiley-Blackwell; 2009. p. 59–84.

41. Gray SR, Abel GG, Jordan A, et al. Visual Reaction Time™ as a predictor of sexual offense recidivism [online first]. Sex Abuse 2013. http://dx.doi.org/10.1177/1079063213502680.

42. Gress CL, Anderson JO, Laws DR. Delays in attentional processing when viewing sexual imagery: the development and comparison of two measures. Legal Criminol Psych 2013;18:66–82. http://dx.doi.org/10.1111/j.2044-8333.2011.02032.x.

43. Knight RA, Sims-Knight JE. The developmental antecedents of sexual coercion against women: testing alternative hypotheses with structural equation modeling. Ann N Y Acad Sci 2003;989:72–85.

44. Knight RA, Prentky RA, Cerce DD. The development, reliability, and validity of an inventory for the Multidimensional Assessment of Sex and Aggression. Crim Justice Behav 1994;21:72–94.

45. Knight RA, Sims-Knight J. Risk factors for sexual violence. In: White J, Koss MP, Kazdin A, editors. Violence against women and girls. Washington, DC: American Psychological Association; 2011. p. 125–72.

46. Miner HM, Robinson BE, Knight RA, et al. Understanding sexual perpetration against children: effects of attachment style, interpersonal involvement, and hypersexuality. Sex Abuse 2009;22:58–77.

47. Mokros A, Dombert B, Osterheider M, et al. Assessment of pedophilic sexual interest with an attentional choice reaction time task. Arch Sex Behav 2010;39: 1081–90. http://dx.doi.org/10.1007/s10508-009-9530-6.

48. Mokros A, Gebhard M, Heinz V, et al. Computerized assessment of pedophilic sexual interest through self-report and viewing time: reliability, validity, and classification accuracy of the Affinity program. Sex Abuse 2012. http://dx.doi.org/10.1177/1079063212454550.

49. Schatzel-Murphy EA, Harris DA, Knight RA, et al. Sexual coercion in men and women: similar behaviors, different predictors. Arch Sex Behav 2009;38: 974–86.

50. Seto MC. The value of phallometry in the assessment of male sex offenders. J Forensic Psychol Pract 2001;1:65–75.

51. Craig LA, Browne KD, Beech A, et al. Psychosexual characteristics of sexual offenders and the relationship to sexual reconviction. Psychol Crime Law 2006;12:
231–43.

52. Nichols HR, Molinder I. Manual for the multiphasic sex inventory. 2nd edition.
Tacoma (WA): Crime and Victim Psychology Specialists; 2000. Available from
Nichols & Molinder, 437 Bowes Drive, Tacoma, WA 98466–70747, USA.

53. Curnoe S, Langevin R. Personality and deviant sexual fantasies: an examination
of the MMPIs of sex offenders. J Clin Psychol 2002;58:803–15.

54. Firestone P, Bradford JM, McCoy M, et al. Recidivism in convicted rapists. J Am
Acad Psychiatry Law 1998;26:185–200.

55. Kingston DA, Bradford JM. Hypersexuality and recidivism among sexual
offenders. Sex Addict Compulsivity 2013;20:91–105.

56. Kingston DA, Firestone P, Moulden HM, et al. The utility of the diagnosis of pedophilia. A comparison of various classification procedures. Arch Sex Behav 2007;
36:423–36. http://dx.doi.org/10.1007/s10508-006-9091-x.

57. Kingston DA, Seto MC, Firestone P, et al. Comparing indicators of sexual sadism
as predictors of recidivism among sexual offenders. J Consult Clin Psychol
2010;78:574–84.

58. Seto MC, Lalumière ML. A brief screening scale to identify pedophilic interests
among child molesters. Sex Abuse 2001;13:15–25.

59. Seto MC, Lalumière ML, Blanchard R. The discriminative validity of a phallometric test for pedophilic interests among adolescent offenders against children.
Psychol Assess 2000;12:319–27.

60. Nunes KL, Babchishin KM. Construct validity of Stable-2000 and Stable-2007
scores. Sex Abuse 2012;24:29–45.

61. Canales DD, Olver ME, Wong SC. Construct validity of the violence risk scale–
Sexual Offender Version for measuring sexual deviance. Sex Abuse 2009;21:
474–92.

62. Seto MC, Harris GT, Rice ME, et al. The Screening Scale for Pedophilic Interests
predicts recidivism among adult sex offenders with child victims. Arch Sex Behav 2004;33:455–66.

63. Leonard RC, Riemann BC. The co-occurrence of obsessions and compulsions
in OCD. J Obsessive Compuls Relat Disord 2012;1:211–5.

64. Letourneau EJ. A comparison of objective measures of sexual arousal and interest: visual reaction time and penile plethysmography. Sex Abuse 2002;14:
207–23.

65. Williams MT, Farris SG, Turkheimer E, et al. Myth of the pure obsessional type in
obsessive-compulsive disorder. Depress Anxiety 2011;28:495–500.

66. Glazier K, Calixte RM, Rothschild R, et al. High rates of OCD symptom
misidentification by mental health professionals. Ann Clin Psychiatry 2013;
25:201–9.

67. Brakoulias V, Starcevic V, Berle D, et al. The characteristics of unacceptable/
taboo thoughts in obsessive-compulsive disorder. Compr Psychiatry 2013;
54(7):750–7.

68. Packard R, Levenson J. Revisiting the reliability of diagnostic decisions in sex
offender civil commitment. Sex Offender Treatment 2006;1(3). Online journal.

69. Wilson RJ, Abracen J, Looman J, et al. Pedophilia: an evaluation of diagnostic
and risk prediction methods. Sex Abuse 2011;23:260–74. http://dx.doi.org/10.
1177/1079063210384227.

70. Doren D, Elwood R. The diagnostic reliability of sexual sadism. Sex Abuse 2009;
21:251–61.

71. Wilson RJ, Pake DR, Duffee S. DSM-5 pedohebephilia, PCD, and sadism diagnoses: reliability in Florida. Paper presented at the 30th Annual Conference of the Association for the Treatment of Sexual Abusers. Toronto, October, 2011.
72. Thornton D, Palmer S, Ramsay RK. DSM-5 pedohebephilia, PCD, and sadism diagnoses: reliability in WI. Paper presented at the 30th Annual Conference of the Association for the Treatment of Sexual Abusers. Toronto, 2011.
73. Abel GG, Becker JV, Cunningham-Rathner J, et al. Multiple paraphilic diagnoses among sex offenders. J Am Acad Psychiatry Law 1988;16:153–68.
74. Bradford JMW, Boulet J, Pawlak A. The paraphilias: A multiplicity of deviant behaviours. Can J Psychiatry 1992;3:104–8.
75. Freund K, Seto MC, Kuban M. Frotteurism and the theory of courtship disorder. In: Laws DR, O'Donohue WT, editors. Sexual deviance: theory, assessment and treatment. New York: Guilford; 1997. p. 111–30.
76. Freund K. Courtship disorder. In: Marshall WL, Laws DR, Barbaree HE, editors. Handbook of sexual assault. New York: Springer; 1990. p. 195–207.
77. Långström N, Seto MC. Exhibitionistic and voyeuristic behavior in a Swedish national population survey. Arch Sex Behav 2006;35:427–35.
78. Långström N, Hanson RK. High rates of sexual behavior in the general population: correlates and predictors. Arch Sex Behav 2006;35:37–52.
79. Kafka MP, Hennen J. A DSM-IV Axis I comorbidity study of males (n = 120) with paraphilias and paraphilia-related disorders. Sex Abuse 2002;14:349–66.
80. Dunsieth NW Jr, Nelson EB, Brusman-Lovins LA, et al. Psychiatric and legal features of 113 men convicted of sexual offenses. J Clin Psychiatry 2004;65:293–300.
81. Fazel S, Sjöstedt G, Långström N, et al. Severe mental illness and risk of sexual offending in men: a case-control study based on Swedish national registers. J Clin Psychiatry 2007;68:588–96.
82. Leue A, Borchard B, Hoyer J. Mental disorders in a forensic sample of sexual offenders. Eur Psychiatry 2004;19:123–30.
83. Marshall WL. Diagnostic issues, multiple paraphilias, and comorbid disorders in sexual offenders: their incidence and treatment. Aggress Violent Behav 2007;12:16–35.
84. McElroy SL, Soutullo CA, Taylor P Jr, et al. Psychiatric features of 36 men convicted of sexual offenses. J Clin Psychiatry 1999;60:414–20.
85. Myers WC. Juvenile sexual homicide. New York: Academic; 2002.
86. Kafka MP. Axis I psychiatric disorders, paraphilic sexual offending and implications for pharmacological treatment. Isr J Psychiatry Relat Sci 2012;49:255–61.

Psychological Treatment of Sex Offenders
Recent Innovations

William Lamont Marshall, oc, PhD, FRSC[a],*, Liam Eric Marshall, PhD[b]

KEYWORDS

- Sex offenders • Psychological treatment • RNR model • Good Lives Model
- Strength-based • Effectiveness • Risk/Needs/Responsivity
- Motivational interviewing

KEY POINTS

- There have been various recent innovations in the psychological treatment of sex offenders.
- Recent innovations include the incorporation of Andrews and Bonta's *RNR Principles*, Ward's "Good Lives Model," and Miller and Rollnick's *Motivational Interviewing*, into a strength-based approach.
- An example of a strength-based treatment program is described and treatment outcome evaluations are summarized.

Abbreviations	
CBT	Cognitive behavior therapy
GLM	Good Lives Model
RCT	Randomized controlled trial
RNR	Risk, Needs, and Responsivity

There have been significant changes in the psychological treatment of sex offenders over the past 15 years in particular. Before that, the field was dominated by the *Relapse Prevention Model*,[1] but emerging evidence had begun to show that excessive adherence to this approach was ineffective.[2] Although some have claimed that retaining some elements of the Relapse Prevention model is valuable,[3] others[4] have completely rejected it.

---

[a] Rockwood Psychological Services, Queen's University, PO Box 50, Inverary, Ontario K0H1X0, Canada; [b] Waypoint Centre for Mental Health Care, 500 Church Street, Penetanguishene, Ontario L9M 1G3, Canada
* Corresponding author.
E-mail address: bill@rockwoodpsyc.com

Psychiatr Clin N Am 37 (2014) 163–171
http://dx.doi.org/10.1016/j.psc.2014.03.006
0193-953X/14/$ – see front matter © 2014 Elsevier Inc. All rights reserved.

RECENT INNOVATIONS

Evidence from other areas of psychological research has shown that avoidance goals are rarely maintained, whereas approach goals are typically sustained over time.[5,6] Consistent with this, the thrust of recent research and theories in clinical psychology strongly indicates that adopting a positive approach to psychological treatment, focusing on building clients' strengths, is more effective than the traditional way of simply eliminating deficits.[7,8] The treatment of sex offenders has begun to assimilate these newer more positively oriented ways of addressing the needs of these clients by adopting Ward's[9] *Good Lives Model* (GLM) and by integrating the motivational style of Miller and Rollnick[10] into the treatment of sex offenders.[11] In addition to these more general shifts in the emphasis of treatment, sex offender programs have, somewhat belatedly, begun to integrate Andrews'[12] *Principles of Effective Offender Treatment.*

Later in this article, an approach to the treatment of sex offenders is described that integrates these recent developments, although the primary aspects of these developments were assimilated into this program (ie, 1991) well before the GLM was described. First, however, a brief description of the 2 primary models is offered, that is, Andrews' Risk/Needs/Responsivity (RNR) and Ward's GLM.

PRINCIPLES OF EFFECTIVE OFFENDER TREATMENT

Andrews and Bonta[12] provided detailed descriptions of a large body of research on which they derived their principles. These studies include the various group-directed meta-analytic studies of the Carleton University, until the recent untimely death of Don Andrews. Such studies show that these principles of effective offender treatment apply equally to offenders of all types, and of both genders, and to adults and juveniles. Hanson and colleagues[13] have demonstrated that these principles apply equally to the treatment of sex offenders and it is clear that, unless they are properly implemented, treatment will not be effective.

Three principles have been shown to be essential. Andrews describes these as risk, needs, and responsivity or RNR. The *Risk* principle is essentially an administrative directive. It accounts for the smallest amount of the beneficial changes induced by treatment, but that should not be taken to mean it is not important. This principle indicates that the greatest benefits (ie, reductions in recidivism) will be obtained by directing treatment at the highest risk offenders. Where resources are limited, only the highest risk offenders should be treated; when greater resources are available, the most extensive and intensive program should be reserved for the highest risk offenders with less time and energy directed at the moderate-risk and lower-risk clients. The *Needs* principle requires treatment to focus on the modification of criminogenic factors, that is, those features of clients that have been shown to predict reoffending but are at least potentially changeable. This principle, when properly applied, accounts for a significant amount of the variance in changes induced by treatment. The *Responsivity* principle, which accounts for even more of the treatment changes, has 2 components: general and specific. Both of these aspects of responsivity reflect the way in which treatment is delivered. Specific responsivity requires therapists to adjust their approach to the unique features of each client: both his enduring features (eg, cultural characteristics, intellectual level, personality style) as well as his day-to-day fluctuations in mood and motivation. Although this is important, it is the general responsivity principle that seems likely to exert the greatest beneficial changes. The core elements of general responsivity include the need for therapists to display the traditionally established features of warmth, empathy, respect, and support while modeling and reinforcing prosocial attitudes and behaviors. When properly enacted, the responsivity principle can, on its own, generate effect sizes in excess of effect size (ES) = 0.23.

Recent research on process factors (ie, features of treatment delivery) in sex offender treatment support and extend Andrews' observations. In detailed studies of sex offender treatment in English prisons, Marshall and his colleagues[14,15] demonstrated that treatment was effective only when therapists displayed warmth and empathy, rewarded clients for each step in the desired direction, and provided guidance as needed. The presence of these therapist features explained between 30% and 60% of the changes brought about by treatment. Of course, the benefits of these character-istics of effective therapists had been demonstrated quite clearly in the general thera-peutic literature over many years.[16] In addition, Drapeau and colleagues[17,18] found that sex offenders reported the behavior of their therapists to be the crucially effective element of their treatment. The behaviors these offenders pointed to as critical were just those that Marshall's studies had shown to produce effective outcomes. Drapeau's clients indicated they wished to be challenged but they said they wanted the chal-lenges to be done in a respectful way; these clients indicated that a confrontational approach made them either withdraw or become hostile. In confirmation of this, studies by Marshall and colleagues described above found that when otherwise warm and empathic therapists engaged in confrontational challenges, all benefits disappeared.

In a final pair of studies examining treatment delivery features with sexual offenders, Beech and colleagues[19,20] found that the group climate created by the therapist was crucial to effective sex offender treatment. Using Moo's[21] well-documented *Group Environment Measure*, Beech demonstrated that it was only when groups were both "cohesive" and "expressive" that sex offender treatment was effective. Cohesiveness describes the whole group supporting one another, encouraging one another for prog-ress, and bonding with each other. Expressiveness occurs when all participants are actively involved in all discussions and where there is freedom of emotional expres-sion. Thus, the limited research on the effective features of the delivery of treatment with sexual offenders is consistent with Andrews' principle of general responsivity.

GOOD LIVES MODEL

Arising initially from Maslow's[22] notion that all humans, whether they are aware of it or not, strive for self-actualization (ie, the realization of their latent potentials), an exten-sive body of research has led to the ideas embodied in what has been described as "positive psychology."[23] Arising from these recent ideas, Ward[9] has integrated various aspects of this research into his GLM, which he suggests provides an approach to the treatment of sex offenders complementary to Andrews' RNR model. The GLM outlines 9 areas of functioning in which people attempt to maximize satisfaction across their lifespan. Most of these areas (eg, satisfactory intimate relations, healthy sexuality) map nicely onto the factors that have been shown in research to be criminogenic deficits among sex offenders.[24,25] Consistent with positive psychology notions, the GLM lends itself very well to a strength-based approach whereby the emphasis is on developing capacities to overcome deficits and offers sex offenders a more hopeful way of looking at their problems. Importantly, the installation of hope has been shown to be crucial to the effective treatment of all manner of psychological disorders[26] and its importance in the treatment of sex offenders has been outlined.[27]

TREATMENT IMPLEMENTATION

Traditional cognitive behavioral therapy (CBT) has dominated treatment programs for sex offenders over the past 40 years. Although applications of CBT to sex offenders evolved as new research became available, there does not appear to be an agreed on model of this approach. Surveys of North American CBT programs for sex offenders have consistently revealed considerable diversity.[28–30] Many of the programs reported in these surveys address several issues that have now been shown to not be criminogenic while neglecting some features that have been shown to be criminogenic. Hanson's excellent series of meta-analyses[13,31,32] has identified criminogenic features of sex offenders and these features should be the focus of interventions. Unfortunately, all too often many of them are omitted from programs while a plethora of noncriminogenic targets are addressed.

The main problematic area of demonstrably noncriminogenic features that treatment providers find difficulty in removing from their program concerns the variety of issues generally subsumed under the rubric "cognitive distortions." Marshall and colleagues[33,34] have written appraisals of the relevant evidence derived from the sex offender–specific literature, as well as from the more general criminologic research, concerning these distortions. In conjunction with Hanson's results, it was demonstrated that issues such as categorical denial, denial of responsibility, minimizations, and other so-called distortions are not criminogenic and should not be addressed in treatment. In conducting training in more than 20 countries, it has been observed that treatment providers are loathe to discontinue using these as treatment targets. In particular, they claim that offenders must take full responsibility for their offense before progress can be made in treatment. This statement is simply not true according to the evidence. It is clear from both criminologic[35] and general psychological research[36,37] that people who make excuses (ie, use cognitive distortions and denial) are not only happier and more healthy than those who readily admit having committed an unacceptable act, but these "deniers" are less likely to repeat the bad behavior. Nevertheless, most sex offender programs resist the evidence and continue to spend needless hours on "correcting" cognitive distortions.

In addition to this resistance, most CBT programs, despite their title, fail to deploy behavioral methods such as therapists self-consciously modeling and explicitly rewarding the expression of prosocial attitudes and behaviors, and they frequently fail to ignore, or otherwise punish, the expression of antisocial attitudes and behaviors. Similarly, CBT programs infrequently, at best, use role-plays, reverse role-plays, and other forms of behavioral practice, as well as between-sessions practice by the clients of the skills they have learned in the therapy room. The latter is essential if generalization of acquired skills and attitudes is to occur. Obviously the aim of treatment is to entrench prosocial behaviors as a dispositional set to be enacted after discharge from treatment. Thus, generalization must be part of the treatment program.

Given these observations, it is perhaps not a surprise that most CBT programs focus on a discourse that is almost exclusively cognitive in content. Indeed, some authors[38] advocate the use of "Socratic" questioning. Andrews and Bonta[12] suggest that, although such approaches are suitable for clients who are above average intelligence and university-educated, most sex offenders seen in prisons and other institutions do not have high levels of education. Consequently, less emphasis on intellectual challenges accompanied by a greater attention to behaviors seems more likely to succeed. Of course, antisocial attitudes and the expression of unhelpful views must be challenged but they must be challenged in any way that is compatible with each client's cognitive skills. In addition, challenges should be respectful, not harsh or demeaning, because the latter diminishes any treatment gains that might otherwise be evident.[17]

Some current sex offender treatment programs have adopted more strength-based and respectful approaches[39–41] deriving in large part from the GLM, and Miller and

Rollnick's[10] Motivational Interviewing. Others, although having absorbed some of these newer styles, still retain a focus on noncriminogenic cognitions and claim that the RNR model is "not prescriptive of treatment practices."[42] Stinson and Becker[42(p6)] claim that the RNR "has not been thoroughly evaluated with sex offender treatment" despite having cited the large-scale meta-analysis of Hanson and colleagues,[13] showing that the implementation of the RNR principles, and only when they are implemented, produce effective treatment results with sex offenders.

From the available evidence, it is clear that to be maximally effective psychological treatment of sex offenders must adhere to the RNR model, integrate the GLM, focus on building strengths, and approach the offenders in a respectful, empathic, and rewarding manner. In the next section, the program the authors have been operating for the past 22 years in a federal prison in Canada is outlined. This approach incorporates all the above features.

AN INTEGRATED STRENGTH-BASED TREATMENT PROGRAM

A brief summary is provided of the critical features of this program because its complete details have been described elsewhere.[41] It is presented to clients in 3 phases: phase 1 is aimed at engaging the clients; phase 2 directs efforts at overcoming criminogenic factors by providing the clients with the skills required to meet their needs in prosocial ways; and phase 3 integrates what the offenders have learned into a future-oriented set of self-management plans consistent with the areas identified in the GLM. One of the problems with most sex offender programs, and indeed with CBT more generally, is a failure to instill in clients the idea that treatment simply moves them along a path toward attaining a better life and that they must continue to develop after discharge. The GLM provides a model that encourages a life course striving toward greater fulfillment.

Because the aim in phase 1 is to win the client's confidence and their engagement in treatment, difficult issues are avoided until these goals are attained. Accordingly, offenders are not asked to provide details of their offenses. They are, however, required to provide a life history covering important events, such as successes and failures during childhood, adolescence, young adulthood, and beyond. From this, the therapist and client collaboratively generate areas where strengths need to be developed (ie, in criminogenic factors such as "relationship skills"). In addition, the offenders are asked to describe disruptions in their lives over the 2- to 3-month period preceding their offense. This description serves to elucidate problematic responses (eg, poor coping) to unexpected difficulties in the period preceding their offense. During phase 1, clients are assisted in bolstering their self-esteem and reducing their sense of shame, both of which are common in sex offenders and both of which block full participation in treatment.[43]

Identified criminogenic targets are addressed in phase 2 using empirically sound procedures. The most common and important criminogenic issues include relationship difficulties, poor self-regulation, sexually deviant interests, sexual preoccupation, and a limited set of problematic attitudes and beliefs. The latter exclude denial, minimizations, excuses, and justifications, all of which, as seen, fail to predict reoffending. More detailed descriptions of these problems, and the effective treatment interventions to develop the requisite skills, are provided in work by Marshall and colleagues.[41]

In the final stage of treatment, all that has been learned in the 2 preceding phases are integrated in phase 3 into a set of future self-management plans. These plans are organized around the GLM and clients are encouraged to continue to work on enhancing their lives after treatment is complete. They are also asked to discuss how they will deal with future problems and avoid placing themselves in risky situations. Finally, they are encouraged to work cooperatively with any supervisors who have been appointed to assist them to remain offense-free.

EFFECTIVENESS OF TREATMENT

Although the influence of treatment on reducing reoffending is the usual way in which effectiveness is determined, there are additional important aspects of effective programs. For example, if most offenders refuse an offer of treatment, then it seems likely that those who accept the offer will be the least problematic. Furthermore, if offenders fail to remain in treatment until they have completed all aspects, they can be assumed to have not lowered their risk to reoffend. Refusal rates reported in the literature range from 7% to more than 80%.[44] The program of Marshall and colleagues[41] has a refusal rate of 3. 8%, but this low rate is partly due to other factors unique to Corrections Canada's prisons, where the program operates. In these settings, it is made clear to the offenders that unless they enter and effectively complete treatment they will not be considered for early release. Furthermore, these programs operate in "program prisons," which means that unless inmates enter and effectively engage in treatment, they may be transferred to a less desirable prison. Not only do these factors influence entry to treatment, they also pressure offenders to complete treatment. Not surprisingly, Marshall's program has high completion rates (ie, 95.8%). Despite these external pressures to enter and complete treatment, programs in other similar Correctional Service of Canada (CSC) institutions have far lower entry and completion rates so the motivational approach of Marshall and colleagues appears to exert an influence.

Debate continues about the effectiveness of sex offender treatment in terms of reduced reoffending. The discussions on one side take the view that effectiveness can only be satisfactorily determined by using a randomized controlled trial (RCT)[45,46] and one side claims that no such study showing positive outcome has yet been described. This claim is not entirely true because multisystemic therapy has been demonstrated to be effective with juvenile sex offenders within an RCT evaluation. Other researchers[47,48] not only point to the difficulties in conducting RCT studies, but also claim there are sound grounds for optimism about effectiveness.

There are now 3 large-scale, soundly designed meta-analyses of treatment outcome with sex offenders.[13,49,50] Although not all programs entering these analyses were shown to be effective, the overall results show clear benefits for treatment. On average, 9% to 11% of the treated groups reoffended, whereas approximately 17% of the matched untreated clients recidivated. Some programs show even more pronounced differences between treated and untreated sex offenders. For example, a study that is in preparation[51] reveals low rates of reoffending (ie, 5.6%) among 535 sex offenders followed for 8.4 years. These results compare favorably with the outcome of a matched group of untreated offenders (approximately 18% recidivism) and a "treatment as usual" group (approximately 11%). The program evaluated in this study is the strength-based approach described above.

SUMMARY

This article has described recent innovations in sex offender psychological treatment that integrates Andrews and Bonta's[12] *Principles of Effective Offender Treatment*, Ward's[9] "Good Lives Model," and Miller and Rollnick's[10] *Motivational Interviewing* into a strength-based approach. An example of a strength-based program is described, which the evidence suggests is effective in reducing sexual reoffending.

The authors recommend that therapists providing treatment for sex offenders incorporate these recent developments in psychological treatment into their programs.

REFERENCES

1. Pithers WD, Marques JK, Gibat CC, et al. Relapse prevention with sexual aggressors: a self-control model of treatment and maintenance of change. In: Greer JG, Stuart IR, editors. The sexual aggressor: current perspectives on treatment. New York: Van Nostrand Reinhold; 1983. p. 214–39.
2. Marques JK, Weideranders M, Day DM, et al. Effects of a relapse prevention program on sexual recidivism: final results from California's Sex Offender Treatment and Evaluation Project (SOTEP). Sex Abuse 2005;17:79–107.
3. Carich MS, Dobkowski G, Delehanty N. No, the spirit of RP is important: a response to Yates & Ward (2009) on abandoning RP. ATSA Forum 2009;21: 1–8.
4. Yates PM. Taking the leap: abandoning relapse prevention and applying the self-regulation model to the treatment of sexual offenders. In: Prescott DS, editor. Knowledge and practice: challenges in the treatment and supervision of sexual abusers. Oklahoma City (OK): Wood'N'Barnes; 2007. p. 143–74.
5. Emmons RA. Striving and feeling: personal goals and subjective well-being. In: Gollwitzer PM, Bargh JA, editors. The psychology of action: linking cognition and motivation to behavior. New York: Guilford Press; 1996. p. 313–37.
6. Gollwitzer PM, Bargh JA, editors. The psychology of action: linking cognition and motivation to behavior. New York: Guilford Press; 1996.
7. Linley PA, Joseph S, editors. Positive psychology in practice. Hoboken (NJ): John Wiley & Sons; 2004.
8. Snyder CR, Lopez SJ, editors. Handbook of positive psychology. New York: Oxford University Press; 2005.
9. Ward T. Good lives and the rehabilitation of offenders: promises and problems. Aggress Violent Behav 2002;7:513–28.
10. Miller WR, Rollnick S, editors. Motivational interviewing: preparing people for change. 2nd edition. New York: Guilford Press; 2002.
11. Prescott DS. Motivational interviewing in the treatment of sexual abusers. In: Prescott DS, editor. Building motivation for change in sexual offenders. Brandon (VT): Safer Society Press; 2009. p. 160–83.
12. Andrews DA, Bonta J. The psychology of criminal conduct. 4th edition. Markham (Ontario): LexisNesis; 2006.
13. Hanson RK, Bourgon G, Helmus L, et al. The principles of effective correctional treatment also apply to sexual offenders: a meta-analysis. Crim Justice Behav 2009;36:865–91.
14. Marshall WL, Serran GA, Fernandez YM, et al. Therapist characteristics in the treatment of sexual offenders: tentative data on their relationship with indices of behaviour change. J Sex Aggress 2003;8:25–30.
15. Marshall WL, Serran G, Moulden H, et al. Therapist features in sexual offender treatment: their reliable identification and influence on behavior change. Clin Psychol Psychother 2002;9:395–405.
16. Marshall WL, Fernandez YM, Serran GA, et al. Process variables in the treatment of sexual offenders: a review of the relevant literature. Aggress Violent Behav 2003;8:205–34.
17. Drapeau M. Research on the processes involved in treating sexual offenders. Sex Abuse 2005;17:117–25.

18. Drapeau M, Korner CA, Brunet L, et al. Treatment at La Macaza Clinic: a qualitative study of the sexual offenders' perspective. Can J Criminal Crim Justice 2004;46:27–44.

19. Beech AR, Fordham AS. Therapeutic climate of sexual offender treatment programs. Sex Abuse 1997;9:219–37.

20. Beech AR, Hamilton-Giachritsis CE. Relationship between therapeutic climate and treatment outcome in group-based sexual offender treatment programs. Sex Abuse 2005;17:127–40.

21. Moos RH. Group environment scale manual. 2nd edition. Palo Alto (CA): Consulting Psychologists' Press; 1986.

22. Maslow AH. Toward a psychology of being. 2nd edition. New York: Van Nostrand Reinhold; 1968.

23. Seligman ME, Csikszentmihalyi M. Positive psychology: an introduction. Am Psychol 2000;55:5–14.

24. Hanson RK, Harris AJ. Where should we intervene? Dynamic predictors of sex offender recidivism. Crim Justice Behav 2000;27:6–35.

25. Mann RE, Hanson RK, Thornton D. Assessing risk for sexual recidivism: some proposals on the nature of psychologically meaningful risk factors. Sex Abuse 2010;22:191–217.

26. Snyder CR. The past and possible futures of hope. J Soc Clin Psychol 2000;19: 11–28.

27. Moulden HM, Marshall WL. Hope in the treatment of sexual offenders: the potential application of hope theory. Psychol Crime Law 2005;11:329–42.

28. Burton DL, Smith-Darden J. North American survey of sexual abuser treatment and models: summary data 2000. Brandon (VT): Safer Society Press; 2001.

29. McGrath RJ, Cumming GF, Buchard BL. Current practices and trends in sexual abuser management: Safer Society 2002 nationwide survey. Brandon (VT): Safer Society Press; 2003.

30. McGrath RJ, Cumming GR, Burchard BL, et al. Current practices and emerging trends in sexual abuser management. Brandon (VT): Safer Society Press; 2010.

31. Hanson RK, Bussière MT. Predicting relapse: a meta-analysis of sexual offender recidivism studies. J Consult Clin Psychol 1998;66:348–62.

32. Hanson RK, Morton-Bourgon KE. The characteristics of persistent sexual offenders: a meta-analysis of recidivism studies. J Consult Clin Psychol 2005; 73:1154–63.

33. Marshall WL, Marshall LE, Kingston DA. Are the cognitive distortions of child molesters in need of treatment? Journal of Sexual Aggression 2011;17:118–29.

34. Marshall WL, Marshall LE, Ware J. Cognitive distortions in sexual offenders: should they all be treatment targets? Sex Abuse in ANZ 2009;2:70–8.

35. Maruna S. Desistance and explanatory style: a new direction in the psychology of reform. J Contemp Crim Justice 2004;20:184–200.

36. Dodge KA. Social-cognitive mechanisms in the development of conduct disorder and depression. Annu Rev Psychol 1993;44:559–84.

37. Schlenker BR, Pontari BA, Christopher AN. Excuses and character: personal and social implications of excuses. Pers Soc Psychol Rev 2001;5:15–32.

38. Mann RE, Thornton D. The evolution of a multisite sexual offender treatment. In: Marshall WL, Fernandez YM, Hudson SM, et al, editors. Sourcebook of treatment programs for sexual offenders. New York: Plenum Press; 1998. p. 47–57.

39. Beech AR, Print B. Strength-based approaches to working with those who sexually abuse: a new paradigm? Paper presented at the 18th Annual Conference of

the National Organization for the Treatment of Sexual Abusers. Cardiff (United Kingdom), September 12, 2008.

40. Bremer J. Building resilience: an ally in assessment and treatment. In: Prescott DS, editor. Risk assessment of youth who have sexually abused: theory, controversy, and emerging issues. Oklahoma City (OK): Wood'N'Barnes; 2006. p. 222–38.

41. Marshall WL, Marshall LE, Serran GA, et al. Rehabilitating sexual offenders: a strength-based approach. Washington, DC: American Psychological Association; 2011.

42. Stinson JD, Becker JV. Treating sex offenders: an evidence-based manual. New York: Guilford Press; 2013.

43. Marshall WL, Anderson D, Champagne F. Self-esteem and its relationship to sexual offending. Psychol Crime Law 1997;3:81–106.

44. Mann RE, Webster S. Understanding resistance and denial, Paper presented at the 21st Annual Research and Treatment Conference of the Association for the Treatment of Sexual Abusers. Montreal (Canada), October 31, 2002.

45. Rice ME, Harris GT. The size and sign of treatment effects in sex offender therapy. Ann N Y Acad Sci 2003;989:428–40.

46. Seto MC, Marques JK, Harris GT, et al. Good science and progress in sex offender treatment are intertwined: a response to Marshall & Marshall (2009). Sex Abuse 2008;20:247–55.

47. Marshall WL, Marshall LE. The utility of the random controlled trial for evaluating sexual offender treatment: the gold standard or an inappropriate strategy? Sex Abuse 2007;19:175–91.

48. Marshall WL, Marshall LE. Treatment of sexual offenders: effective elements and appropriate outcome evaluations. In: Bowen E, Brown S, editors. Perspectives on evaluating criminal justice and correction. London: Emerald Publishing; 2012. p. 71–94.

49. Hanson RK, Gordon A, Harris AJ, et al. First report of the collaborative outcome data project on the effectiveness of psychological treatment of sex offenders. Sex Abuse 2002;14:169–94.

50. Lösel F, Schmucker M. The effectiveness of treatment for sexual offenders: a comprehensive meta-analysis. J Exp Criminol 2005;1:1–29.

51. Marshall LE, Marshall WL, Olver M. A long-term evaluation of a strength-based treatment for sex offenders, in preparation.

Pharmacologic Treatment of Paraphilias

Alessandra Almeida Assumpção, BSW[a], Frederico Duarte Garcia, MD, PhD[a,b],*,
Heloise Delavenne Garcia, MD[a,b],
John M.W. Bradford, MD, DPM, FFPsych, DABFP, FRCPC, CM[c],
Florence Thibaut, MD, PhD[d,e,f]

KEYWORDS

- Sex offender • Paraphilia • Pedophilia • Selective serotonin reuptake inhibitor
- Medroxyprogesterone acetate • Gonadotropin-releasing hormone analogue
- Cyproterone acetate

KEY POINTS

- Paraphilia is a chronic and, in most cases, lifetime disorder.
- The combination of psychotherapy and pharmacotherapy is associated with better efficacy compared with either treatment as monotherapy.
- The gold standard treatment of severe paraphilias in adult males is antiandrogen treatment, especially GnRH agonists.
- Using an appropriate protocol to detect and treat any side effects, antiandrogen therapy constitutes no more or less of a risk than most other psychotropic drugs.
- According to most authors, a minimal duration of treatment of 3 to 5 years for severe paraphilia with a high risk of sexual violence is necessary.
- In juvenile sex offenders, behavioral therapy and SSRIs are the first treatment options.

Disclosure: A.A. Assumpção, F.D. Garcia, H.D. Garcia, J. Bradford, and F. Thibaut have no conflicts of interest.
[a] Department of Psychiatry, INCT-Medicina Molecular, Universidade Federal de Minas Gerais, Avenida Alfredo Balena, 190 Sala 240, Belo Horizonte, Minas Gerais, 30130-100, Brazil; [b] INSERM U1073, Rouen University Hospital, Rouen University, 22 Boulevard Gambetta, Rouen Cx 76183, France; [c] Institute of Mental Health Research, Brockville Mental Health Centre, University of Ottawa, 1804 Highway 2 East, Brockville, Ontario K6V 5W7, Canada; [d] Psychiatry and Addictive Disorders, University Hospital Cochin-Tarnier, 89 rue d'Assas, 75006 Paris, France; [e] Department of Psychiatry and Addictive Disorders, Faculté de Médecine Paris V Descartes, 75000 Paris, France; [f] INSERM U894, Centre des Neurosciences, 2 ter rue d'Alesia, 75000 Paris, France
* Corresponding author. Department of Psychiatry, Avenida Alfredo Balena, 190 Sala 240, Belo Horizonte, Minas Gerais 30130-100, Brazil.
E-mail address: fredgarcia@ufmg.br

Psychiatr Clin N Am 37 (2014) 173–181
http://dx.doi.org/10.1016/j.psc.2014.03.002
0193-953X/14/$ – see front matter © 2014 Elsevier Inc. All rights reserved.

psych.theclinics.com

Abbreviations	
CPA	Cyproterone acetate
DHT	Dihydrotestosterone
DSM	*Diagnostic and Statistical Manual of Mental Disorders*
GnRH	Gonadotropin-releasing hormone
GnRHa	Gonadotropin-releasing hormone analogs or agonists
MPA	Medroxyprogesterone acetate
SSRIs	Selective serotoninergic reuptake inhibitors

OVERVIEW

Paraphilias are sexual fantasies or acts that are deviations from the socially accepted sexual behavior, but may be necessary and, in some cases, sufficient for some people to experience sexual arousal and/or orgasm.[1] The paraphilic spectrum of behavior ranges from nearly normal behavior to being hurtful or destructive to oneself or others. Although paraphilic behavior is not always associated with sexual offences, paraphilic behavior associated with sex offending is a major public health concern. In most cases sex offenders are convicted for child sexual abuse, rape, or sexual assault. Of men born in England and Wales in 1953, 7 in 1000 had a conviction for a sexual offense against a child by the age of 40 years.[2] In more than 90% of cases (99% in Europe), paraphilic sex offenders are males. A recent German study reported 1% of adolescent sex offenders in forensic-psychiatric institutions.[3] Adolescent sex offenders are more frequently observed in North America.

Significant levels of psychiatric morbidity are present in survivors of sexual offences. This was indirectly demonstrated by significant losses of quality of life and productivity and by increased mental health care expenses observed in victims.[4]

Adequate treatment of paraphilic behavior may be effective to prevent acting out and increased victimization, thereby reducing the individual and social burden of paraphilias; it may also improve the quality of life of the paraphilic subject.[1] Recent meta-analyses reported rates of recidivism and risk factors in adult male sex offenders.[5,6] The recidivism rate increased from 15% at 5 years to 27% at 20 years of follow-up. Pedophiles attracted to boys are more likely to reoffend (35% at 15 years) compared with those attracted to girls (16% at 15 years) and to those who offended within their family (13% at 5 years).[5] Some dynamic risk factors were identified, such as sexually deviant thoughts (especially concerning children) and antisocial behavior. Denial, low self-esteem, addictive disorders (mostly alcoholism or drug abuse), and psychiatric comorbid disorders may also increase the risk of recidivism. Dynamic risks may be addressed, and psychotherapeutic treatments may help to improve these factors.

This article reviews current pharmacologic treatment of individuals with a paraphilic disorder. Literature review was performed in MEDLINE PubMed and EBSCO databases using the following key words: "Sex offender," "Paraphilia," "Pedophilia," "Selective serotonin reuptake inhibitor," "medroxyprogesterone acetate," "gonadotropin-releasing hormone analogue," "goserelin," "leuprorelin," "triptorelin," and "cyproterone acetate." All articles published from 1981 to October 2013 in English and French were considered. In addition, Google Scholar database research was performed and the main references and sites were included in the analysis. The references and book chapters on the topic were examined for relevant information and references. This article also considered author's previous publications as a starting point for this review.[1,7–9]

PATIENT EVALUATION

Disclosure is a problem in cases of patients presenting paraphilic thoughts, urges, or behaviors. These patients usually seek help either when the symptoms cause too much anxiety or when they are feeling threatened by legal, labor, or familial issues. Indeed, most of them do not find their sexual fantasies distressing or ego-dystonic enough to voluntarily seek treatment.[10]

A paraphilia by itself does not require immediate psychiatric intervention. A paraphilic disorder is a paraphilia that causes distress or impairment to the individual, or harm to others. Paraphilias themselves are not illegal; however, acting out in response to paraphilic urges may be illegal and, in some cases, could result in severe legal sanctions as occurs in cases of pedophilia.

In the *Diagnostic and Statistical Manual of Mental Disorders* (DSM)-V[11] the category of paraphilic disorders was reshaped to draw a clearer line between atypical human sexual behavior and sexual behavior that causes mental distress to a person or makes the person a serious threat to the psychological and physical well-being of other individuals. Sexual and Gender Identity Disorders Work Group of the DSM-V stated that to be diagnosed with a paraphilic disorder a person needs to: "feel personal distress about their interest, not merely distress resulting from society's disapproval" or "have a sexual desire or behavior that involves another person's psychological distress, injury, or death, or a desire for sexual behaviors involving unwilling persons or persons unable to give legal consent." Before diagnosing a paraphilic disorder in a given sex offender, it is important to recognize that sexual offending may be only secondary to antisocial personality disorders, intoxication by stimulating drugs, dopamine agonist treatments or deep cerebral stimulation in Parkinson disease, a manic episode, delusional disorders, or neurologic diseases. In DSM-V pedophilic disorder criteria remained the same as in DSM-IV TR.

Each sex offender should be carefully examined by at least one mental health professional to make the diagnosis of paraphilic disorders and to adequately diagnose and treat any psychiatric comorbidities. It was recently described[12] that males with paraphilic behaviors associated to an Axis I diagnosis, such as anxiety or affective disorders or substance use disorders are more prone to sexual impulsivity and may get more benefit from pharmacologic treatments. Treatment of comorbid Axis I psychiatric disorders is important but the role of those in acting out of paraphilic subjects remains unclear, except for antisocial personality disorders, which increase the risk of recidivism.

PHARMACOLOGIC TREATMENT OPTIONS

Pharmacologic interventions should be part of a more comprehensive treatment plan including psychotherapy, such as cognitive behavior therapy.[6,8,13,14] Indeed, reducing libido seems to make some offenders with a paraphilic disorder more prone and responsive to psychotherapy.[15]

The pharmacologic treatment of choice essentially depends on[12] the patient's previous medical history, the patient's compliance, the intensity of paraphilic sexual fantasies, and the risk of sexual violence.[8] In subjects with a paraphilia at high risk of victimization, pharmacologic treatment should be used as the first-line treatment option.[8]

No consensus about a minimal duration of treatment was reported. Some authors and international guidelines tend to suggest a minimal duration of 3 to 5 years of antiandrogen treatment in cases of severe paraphilia with a high risk of sexual violence.[8] It is argued that this is the minimal duration necessary for the development of a trustful relationship between the patient and his doctor and for the patient's acceptance of his disorder. However, paraphilias are chronic disorders and a lifelong treatment might be necessary.

Three major classes of medications may be used for the treatment of paraphilic disorders in association with psychotherapy: (1) antidepressants, (2) steroidal antiandrogens, and (3) gonadotropin-releasing hormone analogues or agonists (GnRHa).

A recent German study reported that 16% of all sex offenders in forensic psychiatric institutions were receiving antiandrogen treatment, 11.5% were treated with selective serotoninergic reuptake inhibitors (SSRIs), and 10% with antipsychotic medications.[16] In the United States in 2009, GnRHa were used in, respectively, 13% of all community programs and 15% of all residential programs; medroxyprogesterone acetate (MPA) was used in, 17% of all community and residential programs. In Canada, GnRH agonists were being used in, respectively, 42% of all community programs and 75% of all residential programs as compared with MPA (respectively, 21% and 50%) and cyproterone acetate (CPA) (respectively, 26% and 50%).[17] In more than two-thirds of cases, several medications were used. In Germany, in almost all cases antiandrogen treatment was carried out in combination with psychotherapeutic treatment (cognitive behavioral therapy in 80% of cases).

SSRIs and antipsychotic drugs are not approved for the treatment of paraphilic disorders. Nevertheless, SSRIs were prescribed in more than half of all community and residential programs in Germany and North America.[17]

SELECTIVE SEROTONINERGIC REUPTAKE INHIBITORS

Serotonin inhibits sexual arousal and reduces orgasmic and ejaculatory capacities.[18] Sexual effects of serotonin are receptor-type dependent (ie, the activation of 5-HT_{1A} receptors accelerates ejaculation, the activation of 5-HT_{2C} receptors inhibits ejaculation).[19] Low cerebrospinal fluid concentrations of 5-hydroxyindoleacetic acid, a serotonin metabolite, were reported in men with impulsive aggression.[20,21] Some evidence for an upregulation of 5-HT_{2A} and 5-HT_{2C} was described in one study evaluating eight pedophiles.[22]

Three arguments have been evoked to justify the use of SSRIs in the treatment of paraphilic disorders: (1) the link between serotonin and sexuality, (2) the high rates of anxiety and depressive disorders associated with paraphilias, and (3) the similarities between obsessive-compulsive spectrum disorders and paraphilias.

Although most studies evaluating the use of SSRIs have methodologic flaws, this class of antidepressants has shown good clinical efficacy for the treatment of paraphilic disorders. Patients presenting exhibitionism, compulsive masturbation, and pedophilia without acting out seem to benefit most from SSRIs.[23] SSRIs have been associated with a higher compliance compared with hormonal treatments and have shown good clinical efficacy for the treatment of mild paraphilias.

Fluoxetine and sertraline have been the most studied SSRIs in paraphilias. The efficacy of fluoxetine in the reduction of fantasies and paraphilic behaviors has been described for the treatment of pedophilia, exhibitionism, paraphilia in general, voyeurism, and fetishism. A lack of efficacy was described in one retrospective study using fluoxetine in patients with paraphilias.[1,24] Most of the studies using fluoxetine have used a fast titration until the patient was aware of a significant reduction or a complete disappearance of paraphilic fantasies or urges. The mean dose used was 40 mg (range, 20–80 mg). Treatment was usually interrupted after 4 to 6 weeks in case of insufficient reduction of symptoms.

Sertraline was used in some studies for the treatment of paraphilia and paraphilia-related disorders. A reduction of sexual arousal patterns with suppression of deviant arousal coupled with a maintenance or a relative increase in nonpedophilic arousal in consenting sex with adults have been described.[25,26]

Data supporting the use of SSRIs for the treatment of paraphilias are still scarce, although antidepressants may be an interesting treatment for these disorders even if not formally approved. SSRIs may be prescribed for patients with high level of arousal that cannot be controlled with cognitive behavioral therapies, adding that informed and motivated patients are good candidates. SSRIs could have a specific effect on reducing arousal, independently of their antidepressant efficacy.

SSRIs are probably more effective in paraphilias that resemble or are accompanied by obsessive-compulsive symptoms. SSRIs are primarily indicated for the treatment of mild paraphilias; juvenile paraphilic disorders; or patients presenting comorbidities, such as depression or obsessive-compulsive disorder.[8,25,27]

ANDROGEN-DEPRIVATION THERAPY

Androgens, such as testosterone and dihydrotestosterone (DHT), influence sexual behavior, particularly in men. Androgens enhance the sensitivity of dopaminergic receptors and modulate the effects of $5\text{-}HT_{1A}$ and $5\text{-}HT_{1B}$ receptors on impulsive and aggressive behavior.[28]

The drastic reduction of androgen levels or effects is the cornerstone of hormonal treatment in sex offenders with a paraphilic disorder.[29] According to their mechanism of action, antiandrogen treatments are classified into two classes of medications: steroidal antiandrogens and GnRHa.

STEROIDAL ANTIANDROGEN TREATMENTS

Steroidal antiandrogens, such as MPA or CPA, have progestational activities in addition to their antiandrogenic effects. Through feedback effects on the hypothalamic-pituitary axis that inhibit the secretion of Luteinizing hormone (LH), use of steroidal antiandrogen decreases circulating levels of testosterone and DHT. CPA interferes with the binding of DHT, the androgen that plays the dominant role in androgenic response to androgen receptors and has been shown to block the cellular uptake of androgens.

MPA AND CPA

The use of MPA in sexual offenders with paraphilias was largely described and more than 600 cases have been reported among different studies including 12 case reports, 13 open or controlled studies, and three double-blind and crossover studies comparing MPA with placebo. The oral dosage ranges were 100 to 300 mg/day; parental dosage started from 100 mg given weekly and then was titrated to obtaining a clinical effect on sexual behavior (testosterone levels may be used as an outcome measure). Reduction of sexual behavior and complete disappearance of deviant sexual behavior and fantasies were observed after 1 to 2 months in most studies.[8] However, the risk/benefit ratio did not favor the use of MPA, which is why it was abandoned in Europe.

CPA is predominantly used in Canada, the Middle East, and Europe and is registered in more than 20 countries for the moderation of sexual drive in adult men with sexual deviations. More than 900 men were included in different efficacy studies. Most of the studies reported that CPA given intramuscularly every 1 or 2 weeks (300–600 mg) or orally (100–200 mg/day) during 4 to 12 weeks significantly reduced sexual fantasies and activity in 80% to 90% of subjects. At the end of the follow-up, the average rate of reoffending was 6% after treatment compared with 85% before treatment. Most of the reoffenses were committed by subjects who did not follow the treatment prescription.[8] Depending on dosage, the authors suggested that CPA could be used as a chemical castration agent or as a reducer of sexual drive, allowing erecting ability in case of nondeviant sexual behavior.

For both MPA and CPA informed consent must be obtained. The side effects are related to hypoandrogenism and must be carefully managed medically through frequent follow-up and physical examination. Depressive and emotional disturbances must be evaluated every 1 to 3 months. The effects of MPA and CPA were reversible 1 to 2 months after treatment interruption.[8]

MPA and CPA must not be used before puberty is completed and are not indicated in case of somatic diseases.[8] A specific risk of thromboembolism is observed with both agents. An increased risk of hepatocellular damage is observed with CPA and must be carefully checked.

GnRHa

GnRHa act on pituitary GnRH receptors, interrupting the normal pulsatile stimulation and leading to a desensitization of GnRH receptors. GnRHa indirectly downregulate the secretion of LH (and follicle-stimulating hormone) leading to hypogonadism and thus to a drastic reduction in testosterone levels. During the first weeks of treatment, GnRHa cause an initial testosterone increase (flare-up effect) that theoretically may be associated with increased deviant sexual arousal, fantasies, and behavior. CPA or flutamide may be concurrently used for the first weeks of GnRHa treatment to prevent the behavioral consequences of this flare-up effect.

Side effects related to GnRHa treatment are related to hypoandrogenism, such as hot flushes, asthenia, decreased facial and body hair growth (2%–23%), decreased testicular volume (4%–20%), and mild gynecomastia (2%–7%). They may be specific to the compound use, such as transient pain or cutaneous reaction at the site of injection or a combination of both, nausea, weight gain (2%–13%), blood pressure variations, decreased glucose tolerance, episodic painful ejaculation, diffuse muscular tenderness, sweating, and depressive symptoms. Bone mineral loss should be regularly measured using osteodensitometry in patients receiving GnRHa treatment and treated if necessary.[26] GnRHa treatments should be used after other alternatives have been ruled out or when there is a high risk of sexual violence.

Three GnRHa compounds are currently available: (1) triptorelin, (2) leuprolide acetate, and (3) goserelin. No studies have compared these three compounds.

Triptorelin

Triptorelin is a synthetic decapeptide developed as a pamoate salt (3-mg 1-month formulation; or 11.25-mg 3-month formulation) and recently approved in Europe for the reversible decrease in plasma testosterone to castration levels to reduce drive in sexual deviations of adult men. In total, 75 male subjects (aged 15–57 years) with paraphilia were included in two prospective open studies (N = 41), two retrospective studies (N = 33), and one case report.[26,30–33] In all studies, during GnRHa treatment, no deviant sexual behavior was observed and no sexual offences were committed except for one case. Concurrently, with a rapid and sharp decrease of testosterone and LH levels, reduction of deviant and nondeviant sexual fantasies and behavior was observed and the maximal effect (absence of reported deviant sexual fantasies or behaviors) occurred after 1 to 3 months.

Leuprolide Acetate

Leuprolide acetate was developed as daily intramuscular or monthly depot injections (3.75- or 7.5-mg 1-month formulation; or 11.25- or 22.5-mg 3-month formulation).

Leuprolide acetate efficacy was described in 101 male patients with paraphilic behaviors included in six studies that reported a fast drop of deviant sexual fantasies and behavior. Schober and colleagues[34] have compared behavioral therapy with leuprolide acetate or with placebo in a crossover study including five pedophiles. In three cases, during the placebo phase, deviant sexual fantasies reappeared while testosterone levels were returning to baseline levels.

A pilot study of Moulier and colleagues[35] evaluated changes in brain activation patterns induced by leuprolide acetate in a pedophilic subject in response to pictures of boys compared with an age-matched healthy control subject. Functional magnetic resonance imaging investigations were conducted before leuprolide acetate therapy and at 5 months of leuprolide acetate therapy (associated with psychotherapy and mianserin, 30 mg/day). Before treatment, pictures of boys elicited activation in the left calcarine fissure, left insula, anterior cingular cortex, and left cerebellar vermis. At 5-month treatment, all the previously mentioned brain activations had disappeared and the remaining activated regions were similar to those reported in healthy control subjects. The results suggested that leuprolide acetate decreased activity in regions known to mediate the perceptual, motivational, and affective responses to visual sexual stimuli. In addition, the plasma testosterone level fell to hypogonadal levels.[35]

Goserelin

Goserelin is also a synthetic analogue of GnRH. It was developed as daily intramuscular or monthly depot injections (3.6 or 10.8 mg subcutaneously). Several case reports have described its efficacy in the reduction of paraphilic behaviors.[8]

In the study by Turner and coworkers,[3] side effects were reported in more than 80% of subjects being treated with antiandrogens (either CPA or GnRHa). Most of them were related to the decrease in testosterone levels and are reversible after antiandrogen treatment is stopped. Treatment compliance can be markedly increased if the offender is clearly informed about the possible risks and side effects of antiandrogens, and if he has the feeling that he can freely decide about taking the medication and if he can withdraw from treatment at any time.

SUMMARY

Evidence demonstrates that a combination of pharmacologic and psychotherapeutic approaches may reduce or even suppress deviant sexual behavior in paraphilic disorders. Both SSRIs and antiandrogen treatment efficacy have been reported in populations of sex offenders with paraphilias.

Despite the major social burden of paraphilic behavior, paraphilia disorders still remain under-researched. There is an urgent need for large cohorts of sex offenders and for long-duration follow studies in paraphilic sex offenders.

REFERENCES

1. Garcia FD, Thibaut F. Current concepts in the pharmacotherapy of paraphilias. Drugs 2011;71(6):771–90.
2. Marshall P. The prevalence of convictions for sexual offending, vol. 55. London: Great Britain Home Office Research Development and Statistics Directorate; 1997.
3. Turner D, Basdekis-Jozsa R, Briken P. Prescription of testosterone-lowering medications for sex offender treatment in German forensic-psychiatric institutions. J Sex Med 2013;10(2):570–8.
4. Post LA, Mezey NJ, Maxwell C, et al. The rape tax tangible and intangible costs of sexual violence. J Interpers Violence 2002;17(7):773–82.

5. Hanson RK, Karl R, Harris AJ, Canada CSpepc. La récidive sexuelle: d'une simplicité trompeuse. Ottawa, Canada: Sécurité publique et protection civile; 2004.
6. Hanson RK, Morton-Bourgon KE. The characteristics of persistent sexual offenders: a meta-analysis of recidivism studies. J Consult Clin Psychol 2005; 73(6):1154.
7. Garcia FD, Delavenne HG, Assumpção Ade FA, et al. Pharmacologic treatment of sex offenders with paraphilic disorder. Curr Psychiatry Rep 2013;15(5):1–6.
8. Thibaut F, Barra FD, Gordon H, et al. The World Federation of Societies of Biological Psychiatry (WFSBP) guidelines for the biological treatment of paraphilias. World J Biol Psychiatry 2010;11(4):604–55.
9. Garcia FD, Thibaut F. Sexual addictions. Am J Drug Alcohol Abuse 2010;36(5): 254–60.
10. American Psychiatric Association. Diagnostic and statistical manual of mental disorders: DSM-IV-TR. Washington, DC: American Psychiatric Association; 2000.
11. American Psychiatric Association. Diagnostic and statistical manual of mental disorders: DSM V. Washington, DC: American Psychiatric Association; 2013.
12. Kafka M. Axis I psychiatric disorders, paraphilic sexual offending and implications for pharmacological treatment. Isr J Psychiatry Relat Sci 2012;49(4):255–61.
13. McConaghy N. Paedophilia: a review of the evidence. Australas Psychiatry 1998; 32(2):252–65.
14. Hall RC, Hall RC. A profile of pedophilia: definition, characteristics of offenders, recidivism, treatment outcomes, and forensic issues. Mayo Clin Proc 2007;82(4): 457–71.
15. Murray JB. Psychological profile of pedophiles and child molesters. J Psychology 2000;134(2):211–24.
16. Turner D, Basdekis-Jozsa R, Dekker A, et al. Which factors influence the appropriateness of testosterone-lowering medications for sex offenders? A survey among clinicians from German forensic-psychiatric institutions. World J Biol Psychiatry 2013;1–7 [Epub ahead of print].
17. McGrath RJ, Cumming GF, Burchard BL, et al. Current practices and emerging trends in sexual abuser management. The Safer Society North American Survey, Vol 1. Brandon, Vermont: Safer Society Press; 2009. p. 1–141.
18. Meston CM, Frohlich PF. The neurobiology of sexual function. Arch Gen Psychiatry 2000;57(11):1012.
19. Waldinger MD, Berendsen HH, Blok BF, et al. Premature ejaculation and serotonergic antidepressants-induced delayed ejaculation: the involvement of the serotonergic system. Behav Brain Res 1998;92(2):111–8.
20. Virkkunen M, De Jong J, Bartko J, et al. Relationship of psychobiological variables to recidivism in violent offenders and impulsive fire setters: a follow-up study. Arch Gen Psychiatry 1989;46(7):600.
21. Virkkunen M, Rawlings R, Tokola R, et al. CSF biochemistries, glucose metabolism, and diurnal activity rhythms in alcoholic, violent offenders, fire setters, and healthy volunteers. Arch Gen Psychiatry 1994;51(1):20.
22. Maes M, van West D, De Vos N, et al. Lower baseline plasma cortisol and prolactin together with increased body temperature and higher mCPP-induced cortisol responses in men with pedophilia. Neuropsychopharmacology 2001;24(1):37–46.
23. Adi Y, Ashcroft D, Browne K, et al. Clinical effectiveness and cost-consequences of selective serotonin reuptake inhibitors in the treatment of sex offenders. Health Technol Assess 2002;57:1012–30.
24. Stein DJ, Hollander E, Anthony DT, et al. Serotonergic medications for sexual obsessions, sexual addictions, and paraphilias. J Clin Psychiatry 1992;53(8):267–71.

25. Bradford J, Greenberg D, Gojer J, et al. Sertraline in the treatment of pedophilia: an open label study. Paper presented at the 148th annual meeting of the American Psychiatric Association, Miami, FL, May 20–25, 1995.
26. Hansen H, Lykke-Olesen L. Treatment of dangerous sexual offenders in Denmark. J Forensic Psychiatr 1997;8(1):195–9.
27. Bradford JM. The treatment of sexual deviation using a pharmacological approach. J Sex Res 2000;37(3):248–57.
28. Simon NG, Cologer-Clifford A, Lu SF, et al. Testosterone and its metabolites modulate $5HT_{1A}$ and $5HT_{1B}$ agonist effects on intermale aggression. Neurosci Biobehav Rev 1998;23(2):325–36.
29. Rubinow DR, Schmidt PJ. Androgens, brain, and behavior. Am J Psychiatry 1996; 153(8):974–84.
30. Rösler A, Witztum E. Treatment of men with paraphilia with a long-acting analogue of gonadotropin-releasing hormone. N Engl J Med 1998;338(7):416–22.
31. Thibaut F, Cordier B, Kuhn JM. Effect of a long-lasting gonadotrophin hormone-releasing hormone agonist in six cases of severe male paraphilia. Acta Psychiatr Scand 1993;87(6):445–50.
32. Thibaut F, Cordier B, Kuhn JM. Gonadotrophin hormone releasing hormone agonist in cases of severe paraphilia: a lifetime treatment? Psychoneuroendocrinology 1996;21(4):411–9.
33. Thibaut F, Kuhn J, Cordier B, et al. Hormone treatment of sex offenses. Encephale 1998;24(2):132 [in French].
34. Schober JM, Kuhn PJ, Kovacs PG, et al. Leuprolide acetate suppresses pedophilic urges and arousability. Arch Sex Behav 2005;34(6):691–705.
35. Moulier V, Fonteille V, Pélégrini-Issac M, et al. A pilot study of the effects of gonadotropin-releasing hormone agonist therapy on brain activation pattern in a man with pedophilia. Int J Offender Ther Comp Criminol 2012;56(1):50–60.

Mental Illness and Sexual Offending

Brad D. Booth, MD, FRCPC, DABPN[a,b,c,*], Sanjiv Gulati, MBBS, MRCPsych[a,d,e]

KEYWORDS

- Child sexual abuse • Sexual abuse • Mental disorders • Offenders • Sex offenses
- Paraphilias • Rape

KEY POINTS

- Mentally disordered sexual offenders (MDSOs) comprise a small but significant portion of sexual offenders who require special treatment and resources.
- Psychosis should be stabilized with antipsychotic medications to allow MDSOs to participate in treatment.
- Depression, anxiety, and attention-deficit/hyperactivity disorder can interfere with group treatments and future risk management.
- Dementing illnesses likely provide a special risk factor for those with late-onset offending.
- Ultimately, mental disorders require stabilization before or as part of offender rehabilitation.

Adapted from Booth BD. Special populations: mentally disordered sexual offenders (MDSOs). In: Harrison K, editor. Managing high-risk sex offenders in the community: risk management, treatment and social responsibilities. Devon (United Kingdom): Willan Publishing; 2010; with permission from Taylor and Francis Books, UK.
Disclosures: B.D. Booth: Previous pharmaceutical support (including attending lectures & advisory boards, unrestricted educational grants): Janssen-Ortho Inc, Eli Lilly, Astra-Zeneca, Pfizer; S. Gulati: Previous pharmaceutical support (including attending lectures & advisory boards, unrestricted educational grants): Janssen-Ortho Inc, Eli Lilly, Astra-Zeneca.
[a] Department of Psychiatry, University of Ottawa, 501 Smyth Road, ON K1H 8L6, Canada; [b] Integrated Forensic Program, Royal Ottawa Mental Health Centre, Royal Ottawa Health Care Group, 2nd Floor–Forensics, 1145 Carling Avenue, Ottawa, Ontario K1Z 7K4, Canada; [c] Sexual Behaviors Unit, St Lawrence Valley Correctional & Treatment Centre, PO Box 1050, 1804 Hwy 2 East, Brockville, ON K6V 5W7, Canada; [d] Integrated Forensic Program, Royal Ottawa Mental Health Centre, Royal Ottawa Health Care Group, 2nd Floor–Forensics, 1145 Carling Avenue, Ottawa, Ontario K1Z 7K4, Canada; [e] Assessment & Stabilization Unit, St Lawrence Valley Correctional & Treatment Centre, PO Box 1050, 1804 Hwy 2 East, Brockville, ON K6V 5W7, Canada
* Corresponding author. Integrated Forensic Program, Royal Ottawa Mental Health Centre, Royal Ottawa Health Care Group, 2nd Floor–Forensics, 1145 Carling Avenue, Ottawa, Ontario K1Z 7K4, Canada.
E-mail address: brad.booth@theroyal.ca

Psychiatr Clin N Am 37 (2014) 183–194
http://dx.doi.org/10.1016/j.psc.2014.03.007 **psych.theclinics.com**
0193-953X/14/$ – see front matter © 2014 Elsevier Inc. All rights reserved.

Abbreviations	
ADHD	Attention-deficit/hyperactivity disorder
ECT	Electroconvulsive therapy
GAD	Generalized anxiety disorder
MDSOs	Mentally disordered sexual offenders
NCR	Not Criminally Responsible on Account of Mental Disorder
NGRI	Not Guilty by Reason of Insanity
OCD	Obsessive-compulsive disorder
PTSD	Posttraumatic stress disorder
SORAG	Sex Offender Risk Appraisal Guide
SSRIs	Serotonin-specific reuptake inhibitors

INTRODUCTION

There are now more than 3 times more seriously mentally ill persons in American jails and prisons than in hospitals.[1] Of note, Arizona and Nevada have almost 10 times more mentally ill persons in jails and prisons than in hospitals.[1] With the influx of mentally ill individuals in the criminal justice system, a portion will commit sexual offenses. These mentally disordered sexual offenders (MDSOs) have committed sexual offenses and have comorbid major mental disorders (not including substance or personality disorders). The management plan for MDSOs must include consideration of their illness, and they may need a specialized approach for effective risk management and treatment, both in custody and in the community. This article describes the transinstitutionalization phenomenon, the prevalence of major mental disorders among sexual offenders, and the special considerations and approaches for MDSOs.

TRANSINSTITUTIONALIZATION

Before the 1960s, seriously mentally ill individuals were warehoused in asylums. However, 2 major factors came into play, resulting in an emptying of the asylums, originally termed deinstitutionalization.[2] First, antipsychotic medications became available in the 1950s, providing the first effective treatments for serious mental illness such as schizophrenia and bipolar disorder. Second, the civil rights movement of the 1960s extended to the mentally ill. Institutions with poor conditions were ultimately required to provide a therapeutic environment with appropriate numbers of trained staff. This requirement exponentially increased the cost of providing care for the mentally ill. Furthermore, civil commitment legislation became much stricter. The result of these factors was a dramatic reduction in the number of chronic care beds for the severely mentally ill. For some, this meant significant increases in liberty and true community reintegration. However, for a large number of people with mental illness this meant a lack of appropriate community supports, leaving many without stable housing and without needed supervision. Many of these individuals migrated into the criminal justice system as part of "transinstitutionalization."

The concept of transinstitutionalization is not new, with a historical article from 1939 noting the inverse relationship between beds for the mentally ill and the rates of incarceration in 14 European countries.[3] This trend can clearly be seen in **Fig. 1**. This phenomenon has been observed internationally,[4] including in England and Wales,[5] Canada,[6] and the United States,[7,8] and results in high rates of mental illness among inmates, including sexual offenders.

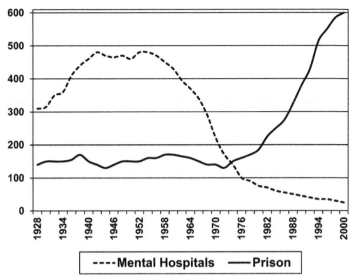

Fig. 1. Rates of institutionalization in the United States (per 100,000 adults). (*Data from* Harcourt BE. From the asylum to the prison: rethinking the incarceration revolution. Tex Law Rev 2006;84(7):1755.)

MENTAL ILLNESS AMONG SEXUAL OFFENDERS

The precise rate of severe mental illness among sexual offenders is not known. However, several studies have examined this issue. Dunsieth and colleagues[9] noted in a sample of 113 sexual offenders that 85% had a substance-use disorder; 74% had a paraphilia; 58% had a mood disorder; 38% had an impulse control disorder; 23% had an anxiety disorder; 9% had an eating disorder; and 56% had antisocial personality disorder. Alden and colleagues[10] demonstrated that psychotic disorders comorbid with personality disorders and substance-use disorders are associated with an increased risk of sexual offending. In another study of outpatients with paraphilias and paraphilia-related disorders (including several sexual offenders), Kafka and Hennen[11] described high rates of mood disorders (71.6%), anxiety disorders (38.3%), and alcohol/substance abuse (40.8%). In yet another study, Ahlmeyer and colleagues[12] found high rates of anxiety, dysthymia, and depression. Within the authors' psychiatric hospital for provincially sentenced offenders in Canada, the rates of serious mental illness is high among sexual offenders, with 43% being diagnosed with depressive disorders, 13% with bipolar disorder, 28% with anxiety disorders, 16% with psychotic disorders, 10% with dementia, 31% with intellectual disability/developmental delay, 42% with alcohol dependence, 38% with substance dependence, 20% with attention-deficit/hyperactivity disorder (ADHD), and 47% with a personality disorder (unpublished data, Booth BD, 2011).

The role of these mental disorders in offending is unclear. Some evidence suggests that mental disorders will increase recidivism and reincarceration in general offenders[13] and in MDSOs.[14,15] However, some evidence suggests that psychotic disorders actually decrease risk in sexual offenders, as noted in one meta-analysis[16] and in the Sex Offender Risk Appraisal Guide (SORAG).[17] It has been argued that mental disorders do not appear to be a criminogenic factor relevant to recidivism.[16,18,19] It is possible that the varying results are a function of whether the underlying mental disorder was detected and appropriately treated; methodological issues in the study design may also be a factor. Regardless, mental disorders require treatment, and some sexual offenders with mental disorders require a modified treatment approach that includes consideration and treatment of their underlying psychiatric disorder.

TREATMENT OF MDSOS

Unfortunately, MDSOs have been unrecognized in the literature as a unique group requiring specialized treatment. As such, the evidence for treatment is limited to clinical experience, derived from evidence-based approaches available for general sexual offenders and the mentally ill. In reality, there is no simple approach. Instead, bio-psycho-social treatment of each MDSO should be tailored to the individual, with the mental disorder being one of many factors that may be relevant to treatment. Treatment should be focused on diagnosis initially, after which targets for treatment should be examined and prioritized for different categories of mental disorders.

The authors' treatment program includes an inpatient unit, which is part of the provincial jail system. The unit is part of a 100-bed psychiatric hospital for provincially sentenced offenders, the first of its kind in Canada. The inpatient interdisciplinary team includes psychiatrists, psychologists, social workers, nurses, substance-abuse counselors, recreation therapists, and vocation staff. During the referral process, residents are flagged by corrections staff as potentially having a mental disorder. When the resident arrives in the institution, he undergoes an initial assessment by psychiatry and nursing, including a comprehensive risk assessment and evaluation by several standardized rating scales. The team prioritizes the treatment needs of the offender. The treatment plan usually includes medication treatment. Also used is the self-regulation group therapy program for sexual offenders described by Marshall and colleagues,[20] including a modified program for developmentally delayed or other cognitively impaired offenders. Anger management and treatment of substance use are also core programs for many residents. At times, severely ill offenders require initial psychiatric stabilization before engaging in group therapy or other modalities focused on criminogenic needs.

Diagnosing MDSOs

The first step in the effective treatment of MDSOs is clarifying the diagnoses and evaluating the potential role of the diagnoses in their sexual offense. However, there are often systemic barriers to achieving this. For example, in the correctional setting MDSOs may have been placed among the general prison population or in protective custody without any screening for mental health issues, and thus may not be seen by a mental health professional or be sent to a treatment facility. Alternatively, if MDSOs do come into a treatment program for sexual offenders, their psychiatric symptoms may be written off as behavioral issues. In the community, MDSOs may be managed primarily by probation and parole officers who may not recognize illness nor have been trained to do so. Alternatively, they may place inappropriate focus on illness as a risk factor, placing significant restrictions on MDSOs.[21] Similarly, community treatment may be provided by individuals with insufficient knowledge about mental illness. Often there is insufficient availability of psychiatric care for sexual offenders.

Ideally, all sexual offenders would be evaluated by appropriately trained individuals for the presence of mental disorders and undergo appropriate treatment of these disorders. Similarly, all individuals who treat and manage sexual offenders should have some training in the diagnosis and treatment of mental disorders. Finally, MDSOs may best be treated in specialized programs that can address both their sexual offense behavior and comorbid illnesses.

Prioritization of Treatment Needs

Once symptoms of mental illness are identified, they must be balanced against other treatment issues, prioritizing these issues and looking at available resources. Symptoms may include psychosis, mood problems, anxiety, substance use, cognitive deficits, attention deficits, and others. MDSOs should be evaluated for the severity of these symptoms and how these symptoms might affect sexual offender treatment (see later discussion). The therapist should prioritize the treatment needs. For example, at times the mental disorder may prevent addressing sexual-offending issues and may require stabilization before treating sexual issues. Symptoms may also be difficult to treat (eg, negative symptoms of schizophrenia) and may require an alteration of regular treatment. At times, optimal treatment may involve treating both issues (the sexual disorder and other mental disorder) at the same time. Alternatively, treatment may simply involve addressing the sexual issues/criminogenic factors and leaving treatment of the mental disorder to others.

Examining the Role of the Mental Disorder in Offending

Once MDSOs' diagnoses are clarified and the treatment needs to be prioritized, individuals involved in the risk management of MDSOs should examine the role that the individual's mental disorder has played in sexual offending. At times, it may be that the mental disorder was causal to the behavior or contributed significantly, providing a clear target for treatment. In other cases, the mental disorder may have been ancillary to the offense, but may become an issue in treatment. Ultimately the role of the mental disorder must be acknowledged and considered in treatment and risk management.

Discussion of comorbid disorders and their potential role in offending should also be introduced into group therapy. Although this approach should always be individualized, there are general issues seen within specific MDSO populations (including psychotic disorders, mood disorders, anxiety disorders, dementing disorder, attention-deficit disorders, substance-use disorders, and personality disorders) that should be brought up for group discussion. Mental retardation and developmental disorders also require a specialized approach, which is discussed by Griffiths and Fedoroff elsewhere in this issue (See also[22]).

SPECIFIC MDSO POPULATIONS
Psychotic Disorders

MDSOs suffering from chronic psychotic disorders, such as schizophrenia, schizoaffective disorder, and delusional disorder, can be some of the most challenging individuals to treat and manage. In the authors' specialized unit for MDSOs, 16% suffer from 1 of these chronic psychotic illnesses. Fewer, but still significant numbers of individuals with psychosis are seen in the outpatient clinic and within the system for MDSOs found Not Criminally Responsible on Account of Mental Disorder (NCR). Despite having profound illnesses, most MDSOs will not be in the NCR system or equivalent system in other jurisdictions, such as Not Guilty by Reason of Insanity (NGRI). For example, in Canada between 1992 and 2005, sexual assault and other sexual offenses accounted for only 4.3% of the total offenses among NCR individuals.[23] Those who do qualify for an NCR/NGRI defense may have their treatment needs regarding sexual offending overlooked, with the treatment team focusing primarily on the mental illness. Treatment should address both the sexual offending and the mental disorder.

Once an MDSO with a psychotic disorder is identified, treatment first involves an analysis of how the illness influenced his actions. Did it contribute directly to the behavior or is it simply an ancillary issue? For example, if a known offender with exhibitionism and schizophrenia had stopped his antipsychotic medications before offending, his sexual offending may have resulted from auditory hallucinations urging his behavior. Issues around medication noncompliance would need to be a part of the treatment plan, and long-acting intramuscular antipsychotic medications may be indicated. In another MDSO with these same illnesses and behaviors, the offending may have been primarily motivated by other issues, such as the presence of a paraphilia.

Once the treating team has an understanding of the role the psychotic illness played in the offense, the individual's current symptoms should be evaluated, including delusions, hallucinations, negative symptoms, cognitive impairment, and disorganization. Do the antipsychotic medications need to be adjusted? For example, an MDSO who is religiously preoccupied may blame "the Devil" for his actions and thus be unable to focus on how his behavior led to offending. Such delusions may respond to adjustments in antipsychotic medications. At other times, chronic residual symptoms that do not tend to respond well to medications, such as cognitive deficits or negative symptoms, might interfere and require alteration of the treatment program. For example, the authors offer self-regulation program sessions in the afternoon to account for sedation from medications, in addition to negative symptoms such as anergy and avolition. Furthermore, those with cognitive deficits and mild developmental delays are entered in a modified self-regulation program, with a slightly simplified approach and more repetition.

At times the treatment of psychosis may supersede the sexual issue, and medication intervention may be required to stabilize psychotic symptoms before commencing therapy. Despite this, residual psychosis is not an absolute contraindication to group therapy. Florid psychosis with active delusions regarding offending would usually be an exclusion criterion for the self-regulation group. The authors have encountered several individuals who were able to effectively address offending behavior despite residual symptoms of their illnesses. It should be noted that leaders of such groups will need to feel comfortable with psychotic content.

When MDSOs with psychotic disorders enter the community, risk management will likely need to involve community supports that are not usually part of most sexual-offender programs. For example, individuals may benefit from living in a group-home or supervised setting where medication compliance can be ensured. Furthermore, individuals may benefit from the support of community outreach programs, such as an assertive community treatment team or other outreach program. Unfortunately, the authors' experience has been that all MDSOs may face discrimination from these outreach organizations. It may prove difficult to overcome the stigma associated with sexual offending. Advocacy and education about MDSOs may be helpful.

Probation and parole officers who supervise MDSOs with psychosis would also benefit from training about these illnesses to better manage risk in the community. For example, when an MDSO has difficulties with conditions imposed by the Court, an evaluation should be done to look at the role that mental illness might be playing. Illness may best be managed through hospitalization and adjustment of medications, rather than pursuing incarceration. Similarly, noncompliance with Court conditions should not automatically be written off as being due to mental illness, and sometimes is more appropriately managed through the Court. Communication between Court officers and the treatment team is important to help address these issues.

Mood Disorders

Mood disorders, especially depression and dysthymia, are highly prevalent in sexual offenders.[9,11,13] Many offenders describe symptoms of depression at the time of the offenses, which may have contributed to their behavior. Furthermore, sexual offenders are frequently vilified in the criminal justice system. Physical assaults, sexual assaults, and scapegoating are not uncommon in prisons,[24,25] particularly for individuals with offenses against children. For many sexual offenders, conviction for a sexual offense will bring the loss of employment, family, friends, status, and financial security. All of these factors likely contribute toward increasing the offender's risk of developing depression. The result is that the offender presenting for treatment and community management may have significant symptoms of depression, which must be considered because they can influence treatment outcome. For example, guilty ruminations can limit gains in therapy if they take a "shame" basis.[26–28] Poor concentration can limit the person's ability to benefit from group therapy and can prevent the assimilation of information between sessions. Low energy can prevent the person from completing homework assignments. Finally, hopelessness can interfere with persons' desire to benefit from treatment if they feel they have nothing to live for. Depressed mood and pessimism can also prove detrimental to the group's milieu and negatively affect other members.

Once again, depression may need to be the target of treatment initially, with consultation by colleagues if required for complex cases. If symptoms are too severe or if the depressed person has any psychotic symptoms, this would be a relative contraindication to beginning group work. If medications are not proving to be effective in treating the depression, electroconvulsive therapy (ECT) may be appropriate in some cases. For example, the authors have sent several clients with severe depression for ECT when treatment with antidepressants has been ineffective. In one case, a client managed in the jail was suffering with undetected depression presented with near catatonia, renal failure, and emaciation. The seriousness of this offender's mental health condition resulted from a general lack of awareness and understanding of mental health issues among correctional staff. Once his illness was appropriately identified and his course of ECT was completed, he was able to engage effectively in the therapeutic process.

Although depression can prevent someone from participating in the group, the authors have also found that the supportive atmosphere of the group can significantly improve depressive symptoms. At times, some individuals will be prioritized to join the group with the goal of addressing guilty ruminations and losses, especially if there are group members with similar losses.

In MDSOs suffering from depression with comorbid paraphilias or hypersexuality, the authors will often offer serotonin-specific reuptake inhibitors (SSRIs) to treat depression, hypersexuality, and paraphilias at the same time.[29–32]

Bipolar illness is less frequent in this population, but again can contribute to offending or be an issue in treatment. Mania and hypomania are usually stabilized before entering group therapy. The potential role of these disorders in disinhibiting the offender and in increasing sexual drive should be part of group therapy discussion.

All individuals with mood disorders may require treatment for these disorders that extends beyond the treatment of sexual offending. Again, resistance from mental health professionals to treat sexual offenders may pose a barrier.

Anxiety Disorders

MDSOs suffering from anxiety disorders are also prevalent,[11,33,34] with social phobia, obsessive-compulsive disorder (OCD), posttraumatic stress disorder (PTSD), panic disorder, and generalized anxiety disorder (GAD) being most relevant.

Anxiety, as part of all of these disorders, can interfere with effective group treatment of sexual offenders. Social phobia may prevent the MDSOs from participating in group discussions and fully benefiting from therapy. Alternatively, they may entirely decline to attend any group therapy. A lack of familiarity with these disorders may cause therapists to misinterpret the lack of participation as resistance to treatment rather than fear of social judgment. Before commencing treatment, it may be necessary to first treat the social phobia with medications or cognitive-behavioral therapy. At the same time, many individuals with less severe social phobia experience the acceptance of the therapy group as extremely validating, and can truly come out of their shells in the context of the group.

Once in therapy, the role of social phobia in offending should be examined during the offense analysis and risk-management planning stages. For example, a socially shy man with pedophilia may have found the acceptance from children comforting, causing him to seek out children for social acceptance. Therapy should include strategies for increasing social acceptance and contact within age-appropriate relationships.

Trauma histories and PTSD appear to be prevalent among MDSOs,[35,36] possibly contributing to offending behavior. Moreover, PTSD may occur in offenders as a result of their offenses.[37,38] Sexual victimization of sexual offenders in prison can also occur[24,25,39] and cause PTSD. Active symptoms of PTSD can complicate treatment by causing uncontrollable anxiety, dissociation, worsening of sleep, and distracting the offender from group discussions. Groups that focus on detailed descriptions of offenses can unmask or worsen PTSD symptoms. However, at times, discussion of trauma issues within the group can assist other group members to see at first hand the effects that their offending may have had on the victim. When discussion of offenses exacerbates PTSD symptoms, it may be necessary to work on trauma issues before entering sexual-offender group therapy. Alternatively, the MDSO with PTSD may need ongoing additional individual support around the PTSD beyond that which can be provided in the group. If not interfering with treatment, trauma issues may best be left to be dealt with at a time when the MDSO's life is more stable.

For individuals suffering from other causes of anxiety, including OCD, GAD, and as part of depression, the symptoms should be evaluated for their role in the offense and potential role in treatment. All individuals may require separate treatment for the anxiety disorder that complements or extends beyond the duration of sex-offender therapy. Once again, issues of stigma may interfere with the individual's ability to obtain such ongoing therapy from other mental health providers.

Attention-Deficit/Hyperactivity Disorder

Adult ADHD is underrecognized and often undertreated.[40] Again, the exact prevalence among sexual offenders is not known. However, in a consecutive group of outpatients in a sexual behaviors clinic, the retrospective rate of childhood ADHD was 36%.[11] In addition, childhood ADHD was associated with paraphilic disorders.[41] In the authors' inpatient unit, the adult ADHD rate among MDSOs is 20%. Symptoms of ADHD, such as impulsivity and difficulty evaluating consequences, may contribute to offending behavior or interfere with group treatment.

In group treatment, residual hyperactive and impulsive symptoms may interfere with the person's ability to interact in the group. He may interrupt frequently, talk too much, or blurt out derogatory comments to other group members. In addition, he may have a limited ability to remain seated and quiet for the duration of the group session. Deficits in attention can limit his ability to benefit from other group members' comments. He may also have difficulties completing group assignments or organizing an effective risk-management plan.

Given the potential role of ADHD in offending and in interfering with group therapy in addition to the general impairments caused by untreated ADHD, MDSOs with ADHD should be offered pharmacological treatment. Interestingly methylphenidate, a psychostimulant used in the treatment of ADHD, was added to augment SSRI treatment in a single study of 26 men with paraphilias or paraphilia-related disorders.[42] The addition of methylphenidate in this study was associated with further significant decreases in total sexual outlet and average time spent per day in paraphilia/paraphilia-related behavior. These gains appeared to be independent of the presence of ADHD. This finding suggests a possible additional benefit to prescribing methylphenidate for ADHD treatment in individuals with paraphilias. Of note, this was a small study that has not been replicated.

Despite the potential benefits of ADHD treatment, sexual offenders have high rates of substance abuse,[15,34,43] and there thus is a potential for diversion or abuse of these medications. As such, stimulants should be prescribed in a slow-release form (such as OROS methylphenidate). Alternatively, nonstimulant treatment of ADHD (eg, atomoxetine or bupropion) may be preferred.

Dementing Disorders

Dementing disorders, such as Alzheimer dementia and multi-infarct dementia, are also becoming increasingly prevalent among MDSOs. As noted by Fazel and colleagues,[44] about half of male prisoners older than 59 years are incarcerated for sexual offenses, making the possibility of dementia in the sexual-offender population realistic. However, dementia was an infrequent diagnosis in his group. In the authors' facility, dementia constitutes approximately 10% of the population; several MDSOs with dementia have been found permanently Unfit to Stand Trial and are managed in the NCR/NGRI system. Regardless of the rates, the MDSO with dementia often has specialized treatment needs and risk-management considerations.

As with other MDSOs, the initial step is diagnostic clarification. One must attempt to confirm the cause of the dementia, the prognosis, the deficits present, and the treatment needs of the offender. The diagnostic workup can include neuropsychological testing, cognitive testing, magnetic resonance imaging/computed tomography of the head, and blood testing, such as a vitamin B_{12} level and a syphilis screen (VDRL test).

Once the diagnosis is clarified, the role of dementia in the index offenses should be established. MDSOs with dementia may come to attention as part of a current offense or from offenses committed years before. Although, statistically, frontal lobe disinhibition in the elderly does not appear to be an important factor in sexual offending,[44] it nonetheless may have played an important role for an individual offender. Was an underlying paraphilia acted on because of reduced inhibition from a dementia? Was this a de novo offense that appears to be a personality change (as can occur in frontal lobe dementia)? Moreover, individuals with dementia are more susceptible to developing delirium: was the offense part of a delirium? At times, nursing homes or the legal system may misinterpret sexual behaviors that occur as part of dementia as intentional and illegal behaviors.

Dementia frequently becomes relevant for treatment and risk management. The MDSO with dementia may have difficulties remembering the offense, which limits the role of treatments that focus on detailed analysis and discussion of the offense. Memory deficits may also interfere with remembering group discussions beyond the session or between sessions. If the person is able to learn and retain information, it is likely worthwhile to have him in the group. However, individuals with moderate and severe dementia would be unlikely to significantly benefit from these approaches.

In some MDSOs with dementia, risk management may need to focus on other issues. For example, treatment may focus on slowing further cognitive decline through the use of acetylcholinesterase inhibitors or through control of hypertension and hypercholesterolemia. Reversible causes of dementia, such as nutritional deficits and tertiary syphilis, should be treated. Treatment may also entail pharmacological interventions aimed directly at sexual offending, such as SSRIs or antiandrogen therapy. However, given the high rates of physical illness, consultation from other medical colleagues may be required before initiating such therapies.

Ultimately, risk management of the MDSO with dementia may need to focus on appropriate housing and supervision in a structured environment. For individuals with offenses against children, there may be a theoretically increased risk in some residences; for example, through having access to children who come to visit grandparents in a nursing home. Usually this risk can be entirely controlled through education of the staff and appropriate supervision. Unfortunately, again owing to stigma, the more common problem is persuading nursing homes and other residences for the elderly to accept an MDSO with dementia. Usually education and close partnerships with these institutions will help.

SUMMARY

Sexual offenders suffering from mental disorders are common, and require appropriate diagnosis and treatment of their mental disorders to optimize treatment outcomes. Often these mental disorders play a role in sexual offending, and require special attention so as to provide appropriate treatment and manage risk. Individuals involved in the care and supervision of sexual offenders should be aware of mental illness and its potential impact on treatment.

REFERENCES

1. Torrey EF, Kennard AD, Eslinger D, et al. More mentally ill persons are in jails and prisons than hospitals: a survey of the States. Alexandria, VA: National Sheriffs' Association, Treatment Advocacy Center; May, 2010. Available at: www.treatmentadvocacycenter.org/storage/documents/final_jails_v_hospitals_study.pdf.
2. Talbott JA. Deinstitutionalization: avoiding the disasters of the past. Psychiatr Serv 2004;55(10):1112–5.
3. Penrose LS. Mental disease and crime: outline of a comparative study of European statistics. Br J Med Psychol 1939;18:1–15.
4. Fakhoury W, Priebe S. The process of deinstitutionalization: an international overview. Curr Opin Psychiatr 2002;15(2):187–92.
5. Gunn J. Future directions for treatment in forensic psychiatry. Br J Psychiatr 2000; 176(4):332–8.
6. Sealy P, Whitehead PC. Forty years of deinstitutionalization of Psychiatric Service in Canada: an empirical assessment. Can J Psychiatry 2004;49(4):249–57.
7. Harcourt BE. From the asylum to the prison: rethinking the incarceration revolution. Tex Law Rev 2006;84(7):1751–86.
8. Konrad N. Prisons as new asylums. Curr Opin Psychiatr 2002;15(6):583–7.
9. Dunsieth NW Jr, Nelson EB, Brusman-Lovins LA, et al. Psychiatric and legal features of 113 men convicted of sexual offenses. J Clin Psychiatry 2004;65(3): 293–300.
10. Alden A, Brennan P, Hodgins S, et al. Psychotic disorders and sex offending in a Danish birth cohort. Arch Gen Psychiatry 2007;64(11):1251–8.

11. Kafka MP, Hennen J. A DSM-IV Axis I comorbidity study of males (n = 120) with paraphilias and paraphilia-related disorders. Sex Abuse 2002;14(4):349–66.
12. Ahlmeyer S, Kleinsasser D, Stoner J, et al. Psychopathology of incarcerated sex offenders. J Personal Disord 2003;17(4):306–18.
13. Baillargeon J, Binswanger IA, Penn JV, et al. Psychiatric disorders and repeat incarcerations: the revolving prison door. Am J Psychiatry 2009;166(1):103–9.
14. Fazel S, Sjöstedt G, Långström N, et al. Severe mental illness and risk of sexual offending in men: a case-control study based on Swedish national registers. J Clin Psychiatry 2007;68(4):588–96.
15. Langstrom N, Sjostedt G, Grann M. Psychiatric disorders and recidivism in sexual offenders. Sex Abuse 2004;16(2):139–50.
16. Bonta J, Law M, Hanson K. The prediction of criminal and violent recidivism among mentally disordered offenders: a meta-analysis. Psychol Bull 1998; 123(2):123–42.
17. Quinsey VL, Harris GT, Rice ME, et al. Violent offenders: appraising and managing risk. Washington, DC: American Psychological Association; 1998.
18. Phillips HK, Gray NS, MacCulloch SI, et al. Risk assessment in offenders with mental disorders: relative efficacy of personal demographic, criminal history, and clinical variables. J Interpers Violence 2005;20(7):833–47.
19. Bonta J, Blais B, Wilson HA. The prediction of risk for mentally disordered offenders: a quantitative synthesis 2013-01. In: P.S. Canada, editor. Ottawa (Canada): Public Safety Canada; 2013. Available at: http://www.publicsafety.gc.ca/cnt/rsrcs/pblctns/prdctn-rsk-mntlly-dsrdrd/prdctn-rsk-mntlly-dsrdrd-eng.pdf.
20. Marshall WL, Marshall LE, Serran GA, et al. Treating sexual offenders: an integrated approach. New York: Routledge; 2006.
21. Louden JE, Skeem JL. How do probation officers assess and manage recidivism and violence risk for probationers with mental disorder? An experimental investigation. Law Hum Behav 2013;37(1):22–34.
22. van Horn J, Mulder J, Kusters I. Intellectually disabled sexual offenders: subgroup profiling and recidivism after outpatient treatment. In: Harrison K, editor. Devon (United Kingdom): Willan Publishing; 2010.
23. Latimer J. The review board systems in Canada: overview of results from the mentally disordered accused data collection study. In: Department of Justice, editor. 2006. Ottawa (Canada): p. 1–52. Available at: http://www.justice.gc.ca/eng/rp-pr/csj-sjc/jsp-sjp/rr06_1/rr06_1.pdf.
24. Dumond R. Confronting America's most ignored crime problem: the Prison Rape Elimination Act of 2003. J Am Acad Psychiatry Law 2003;31(3):354–60.
25. Jones TR, Pratt TC. The prevalence of sexual violence in prison: the state of the knowledge base and implications for evidence-based correctional policy making. Int J Offender Ther Comp Criminol 2008;52(3):280–95.
26. Proeve M, Howells K. Shame and guilt in child sexual offenders. Int J Offender Ther Comp Criminol 2002;46(6):657–67.
27. Bumby KM, Marshall WL, Langton CM. A theoretical model of the influences of shame and guilt on sexual offending. In: Schwartz BK, editor. The sex offender: theoretical advances, treating special populations and legal developments. Thousand Oaks (CA): Sage; 1999. p. 1–12.
28. Hudson SM, Ward T, Marshall WL. The abstinence violation effect in sex offenders: a reformulation. Behav Res Ther 1992;30(5):435–41.
29. Greenberg D, Bradford JM. Treatment of the paraphilic disorders: a review of the role of the selective serotonin reuptake inhibitors. Sex Abuse 1997;9: 349–61.

30. Bradford JM. The neurobiology, neuropharmacology, and pharmacological treatment of the paraphilias and compulsive sexual behaviour. Can J Psychiatry 2001; 46(1):26–34.
31. Hill A, Briken P, Kraus C, et al. Differential pharmacological treatment of paraphilias and sex offenders. Int J Offender Ther Comp Criminol 2003;47(4):407–21.
32. Adi Y, Ashcroft D, Browne K, et al. Clinical effectiveness and cost-consequences of selective serotonin reuptake inhibitors in the treatment of sex offenders. Health Technol Assess 2002;6(28):1–66.
33. Hoyer J, Kunst H, Schmidt A. Social phobia as a comorbid condition in sex offenders with paraphilia or impulse control disorder. J Nerv Ment Dis 2001;189(7):463–70.
34. Raymond NC, Coleman E, Ohlerking F, et al. Psychiatric comorbidity in pedophilic sex offenders. Am J Psychiatry 1999;156(5):786–8.
35. McMackin RA, Leisen MB, Cusack JF, et al. The relationship of trauma exposure to sex offending behavior among male juvenile offenders. J Child Sex Abus 2002; 11(2):25–40.
36. Marshall WL, Marshall LE. The origins of sexual offending. Trauma Violence Abuse 2000;1(3):250–63.
37. Gray NS, Carman NG, Rogers P, et al. Post-traumatic stress disorder caused in mentally disordered offenders by the committing of a serious violent or sexual offence. J Forensic Psychiatr Psychol 2003;14(1):27.
38. Crisford H, Dare H, Evangeli M. Offence-related posttraumatic stress disorder (PTSD) symptomatology and guilt in mentally disordered violent and sexual offenders. J Forensic Psychiatr Psychol 2008;19(1):86–107.
39. Wolff NP, Blitz CL, Shi JM. Rates of sexual victimization in prison for inmates with and without mental disorders. Psychiatr Serv 2007;58(8):1087–94.
40. Barkley RA, Brown TE. Unrecognized attention-deficit/hyperactivity disorder in adults presenting with other psychiatric disorders. CNS Spectr 2008;13(11): 977–84.
41. Kafka MP, Prentky RA. Attention-deficit/hyperactivity disorder in males with paraphilias and paraphilia-related disorders: a comorbidity study. J Clin Psychiatry 1998;59(7):388–96.
42. Kafka MP, Hennen J. Psychostimulant augmentation during treatment with selective serotonin reuptake inhibitors in men with paraphilias and paraphilia-related disorders: a case series. J Clin Psychiatry 2000;61(9):664–70.
43. Kafka MP, Prentky RA. Preliminary observations of DSM-III-R axis I comorbidity in men with paraphilias and paraphilia-related disorders. J Clin Psychiatry 1994; 55(11):481–7.
44. Fazel S, Hope T, O'Donnell I, et al. Psychiatric, demographic and personality characteristics of elderly sex offenders. Psychol Med 2002;32(2):219–26.

Persons with Intellectual Disabilities and Problematic Sexual Behaviors

Dorothy M. Griffiths, CM, OOnt, PhD[a],*, Paul Fedoroff, MD[b]

KEYWORDS

- Intellectual disability • Sexual deviance • Counterfeit deviance • Paraphilia

KEY POINTS

- People with intellectual disabilities and problematic sexual behaviors have the same rights as those without intellectual disability. Often their needs are more complex. Often they require more support. They are typically more vulnerable.
- People with intellectual disabilities have the same range of sexual interests and behaviors as the general public.
- Treatment programs that start with the preceding premises are highly successful.

Abbreviations	
DM-ID	Diagnostic Manual–Intellectual Disability
GnRH	Gonadotropin releasing hormone agonists
IM	Intramuscular injection

INTRODUCTION
Nature of Problem

According to the American Association for Intellectual and Developmental Disability,[1] intellectual disability is defined by the presence of challenges originating before the age of 18 years in both mental capacity (noted by an intelligence quotient of less than 75) and adaptive behavior that affects activities of everyday life. Approximately

Disclosure: The authors do not benefit financially from the content of this article.
[a] International Dual Diagnosis Certificate Programme, Department of Child and Youth Studies, Centre of Applied Disability Studies, Brock University, 500 GlenRidge Avenue, St Catharines, Ontario L2S 3A1, Canada; [b] Sexual Behaviours Clinic, Division of Forensic Psychiatry, Institute of Mental Health Research, Royal Ottawa Mental Health Centre, University of Ottawa, 1145 Carling Avenue, Ottawa, Ontario K1Z 7K4, Canada
* Corresponding author.
E-mail address: dgriffiths@brocku.ca

Psychiatr Clin N Am 37 (2014) 195–206
http://dx.doi.org/10.1016/j.psc.2014.03.005
0193-953X/14/$ – see front matter © 2014 Elsevier Inc. All rights reserved.

2% to 3% of the population has an intellectual disability. However, it has been identified that 30.7% of a study group of prisoners had intellectual disabilities.[2] The main offenses committed by persons with intellectual disabilities leading to criminal charges are sexual offenses, arson, and violent conduct.[3,4]

The increased rates of sexual offenses by people with intellectual disabilities may be caused by several factors. The proportional overrepresentation may relate in part to increased vulnerabilities associated with the intellectual disability, such as impaired judgment or lack of adaptive abilities; or the risk factors potentially associated with the lifestyle of a person with an intellectual disability, including poverty, clustered living, lack of education, and abusive experiences.[5] Firth[6] hypothesized that, because of the high rates of sexual abuse experienced by persons with intellectual disabilities, they may be more likely to commit a sexual offense at a later point in their life. However the rates may reflect the increased likelihood that a person with intellectual disability will be arrested, confess to a crime they may or may not have committed, incriminate themselves, waive their rights, or fail to plea bargain or appeal a judgment.[7-10] They also represent a segment of the population that is likely to be financially unable to obtain and afford appropriate legal assistance in their interactions with the criminal-justice system.[11]

However, other investigators have suggested that persons with intellectual disabilities are often excluded from prosecution because of diversion programs that place them in alternative settings that are outside the justice system.[12,13] As such, the true statistics and the reasons for them continue to be highly controversial.

DIAGNOSTIC ISSUES

The DSM-5 defines paraphilic disorders as paraphilias that meet category B criteria which are either as having acted on paraphilic sexual urges (in the case of illegal sex acts) and/or "the sexual urges or fantasies cause clinically significant distress or impairment in social, occupational, or other important areas of functioning". Assessment of how much a paraphilia specifically impacts on the social, occupation and other areas of functioning in people with intellectual disabilities often requires close collaboration with care providers who can assist in answering questions about the impact of the paraphilic interests and behaviours.

Day[12] divided sexual transgressions observed in persons with intellectual disabilities into 2 categories. The first group commits sexual transgressions only, whereas the second group presents with a range of offenses including those that are sexual. Members of the group that have committed a sexual offense only usually engage in offensive behaviors that are more naive or nuisance offenses, are less serious, and are less specific to choice of victim type. Members of this group typically have mild intellectual disability, with no evidence of mental disorder, specific brain damage, or generalized problem behaviors. In contrast, the second group shows a higher incidence of sociopathic and challenging behaviors, and brain damage. Their sexual offenses are both more specific to victim and more persistent. The second group was also described by Day[12] as being less sexually naive.

In a more recent study, Lunsky and colleagues[14] compared the sexual knowledge and attitudes of 48 men with intellectual disabilities, who had sexually offended, with a matched sample of nonoffenders with intellectual disabilities. Among the offender group there were 2 types of offenders. Type 1 offenders were described as "paedophiles, rapists or having engaged in repeated sexual assaults"; type 2 offenders had engaged in behaviors such as, "inappropriate touching, public exhibitionism or public masturbation"[14(p76)]. Their study showed that the type I offenders had significantly more sexual knowledge than the nonoffender group. However, the type II offenders showed the same degree of sexual knowledge as the group of persons with intellectual disabilities who had never offended. The investigators concluded that the study supported Day's[12] observation that there may be 2 types of offenders who have intellectual disabilities.

Day[12] suggested that, although rare, paraphilias can occur in the population of persons with intellectual disability. Clinicians need to cautiously evaluate the presenting offense in terms of its nature and severity. This caution had been elaborated on earlier by Hingsburger and colleagues[15] who posited the theory of counterfeit deviance (in recent years there has been increased interest in researching aspects of the theory of counterfeit deviance). However, many of the articles have been based on a misunderstanding of the original thesis, which was printed in a journal that has since been discontinued. The theory of counterfeit deviance was therefore revisited and expanded by Griffiths and colleagues in a 2013 article published in the *Journal of Applied Research in Intellectual Disabilities*. They presented 14 cases showing different hypotheses to explain the sexually offending behavior. Three of the cases were examples of paraphilias unlikely to lead to illegal behavior, such as a shoe fetish; a paraphilia that could lead to an illegal act such as pedophilia; and so-called hypersexuality. The remaining 11 cases represented examples that phenomenologically seemed to be examples of sexual deviance but that, on closer examination, lacked the elements of sexual urges or fantasies to warrant them being categorized as being caused by sexual deviance or diagnosed as a paraphilic disorder. The article noted that behaviors were often associated with restricted or atypical life experiences, such as a lack of privacy, maladaptive learning history, pathologic modeling, inappropriate partner selection or courtship, or lack of moral or sexual education.

A classic example, presented by Hingsburger[16] involved a man who had lived in a sexually punitive institutional environment. He had been diagnosed with coprophilia. However, on reexamination, it was learned that the person used feces to masturbate not because of a sexualized association with feces but as a substitute for lubricant in which to facilitate a more expedient ejaculation. In this case, the person was living in an environment that made his unconventional behavior expeditious. However, because he was not sexually aroused by feces and was eager to learn an alternative approach to reach satisfaction, he did not meet diagnostic criteria for coprophilia.

The concept of counterfeit deviance was listed as one of the factors to consider before diagnosing a paraphilic disorder in persons with intellectual disabilities in the Diagnostic Manual–Intellectual Disability (DM-ID,[17]) which was written as a companion manual for clinicians using the Diagnostic and Statistical Manual of Mental Disorders criteria to diagnose persons with intellectual disabilities. The DM-ID[18(p427)] states:

A careful differential diagnosis, based on an evaluation of the individual's environment, sociosexual knowledge and attitudes, learning experiences, partner selection, courtship skills, and biomedical influences, is required to differentiate a Paraphilia from counterfeit deviance.

The manual also noted that the assessment of persons with intellectual disabilities may require both special caution and the application of different assessment tools, especially to ensure appropriate diagnosis of paraphilic disorders. When a person with an intellectual disability is referred for assessment for an offense, a test of intelligence is often administered to determine the level of cognitive functioning and to ensure that the individual meets the criteria for intellectual disability. Although this test may provide information that may assist the clinician concerning the relative strengths and weakness of the person's learning abilities, the application of a single source of information, such as mental age, should not be misapplied as predictive of the individual's functioning relative to sexual knowledge or interest and does not account for the life experiences of the individual. An adult with the mental age of a child still has the life experiences, and the physical development, of an adult.[18]

The DM-ID (currently undergoing revision to respond to the changes in the DSM that were made in 2013)[18] noted that the DSM Fourth Edition, Text Revision criteria for the paraphilia applies generally to this population with the following cautions:

1. When considering a diagnosis of a paraphilia, clinicians should rule out the potentially rival hypothesis of counterfeit deviance, particularly for those who are less verbal.
2. Diagnosis of a paraphilia should be made only after elimination of the possibility that the behavior may represent:
   - Behaviors learned from atypical experiences caused by institutional living or abuse
   - A traumagenic reenactment
   - A lack of knowledge such as the difference between private and public
   - The sequela of a medical condition such as a genetic syndrome
   - Inadequate exposure to habilitative life experiences, including sexual experiences
   - Inability to accurately identify age of self, age of a child, or age of an appropriate sexual partner

OVERVIEW OF EVALUATION

Evaluations should be conducted from a combination of biopsychosocial perspectives.

A paraphilia might reflect the interactive effects of anatomic or physiologic influences (ie, physical, neurologic, biomedical, sensory, or mental health influences); psychological characteristics (ie, cognitions, motivational features, communication skills, emotional expressions, anger management skills, or coping skills); and socioenvironmental influences (eg, physical environmental features and social interactions).[17(p435)]

Biomedical

Persons with intellectual disabilities are a heterogeneous group, consisting of people with a large range of problems, syndromes, and diseases. Some intellectual disabilities are genetically determined, others are caused by medical, environmental, or accidental factors. For others the cause is unknown. Knowledge of the syndrome can, in some cases, provide valuable information regarding nature of the sexually deviant act or the factors that may have contributed to the expression of the act. For example, persons with Smith-Magenis syndrome engage in polyembolokoilamania, which can be mistaken as a sexually motivated behavior when it involves insertion of unusual objects in an orifice such as the anus; persons with Tourette syndrome may touch themselves or others in a seemingly sexual way because of motor tics; or persons with Williams syndrome may engage in disinhibited social interactions.

Persons with intellectual disabilities are 2 to 4 times more likely to have concurrent psychiatric disorders, many of which are unidentified.[19] The presence of intellectual disability often diagnostically overshadows the mental health problem and, as such, they more often fail to receive appropriate diagnostic services or treatment.[20,21] Fedoroff and colleagues[22] noted that, as treatment progresses, previously masked disorders may be revealed. Thus, in addition to evaluation of the presenting sexual problem, there is the need for comprehensive evaluation and treatment of medical and psychiatric disorders.

Psychological

Some risk factors that have been correlated with the paraphilias are more likely to be present in persons with intellectual disabilities. These risk factors include challenges in attachment,[23] positive sociosexual skill development,[24] and repressive or abusive early experiences.[25,26] Some persons with intellectual disabilities who live in congregate settings, in which their sexuality is highly controlled or punished, have been noted to develop erotophobia that includes negative reactions to anything sexual, including anger and even fear of their own genitals.[25] People with intellectual disabilities are 1.5 times more likely to be at risk of sexual abuse.[26] For some individuals their first and perhaps only sexual experience may have been abusive. It is important to remember that disclosure of personal traumatic experience is difficult at any time. It is even more difficult for individuals undergoing the additional stress of a court-ordered assessment. These problems are compounded if the person has language or intellectual deficits. A decision to not disclose past abuse is even more unlikely because it is often labeled as an attempt to avoid responsibility for the current offense.

Griffiths and Fedoroff[27] described how the cognitive challenges of the individual can increase the possibility of nonparaphilic activities seeming to be abnormal. One case involved a young man who repeatedly masturbated in the common room of a group home when a particular woman was present. Attempts to redirect him to a private place failed. Staff labeled him as an exhibitionist. A rival hypothesis to exhibitionism (a condition in which the person is aroused by being seen by a stranger) was posed. Perhaps the man required the assistance of visual stimulation to assist him to become aroused. The hypothesis was tested by providing him with legal erotic materials that he could view in private. The problematic behavior quickly resolved. In this case the man's problem was not exhibitionism but an inability to fantasize. The public masturbation was resolved by providing him with a way to masturbate in private.

Socioenvironmental

Day[28] posited that the repressive and restrictive learning environments and attitudes that surround the sexuality of persons with intellectual disabilities may be an important factor in the presentation of problematic sexual behaviors. Clinical examples have been presented in the literature of individuals who, after repeated punishment of consenting relationships with age-appropriate partners, turned to children as a source of sexual pleasure[15] or resorted to engaging in quick nonconsensual sexual acts that they hoped would go undetected by staff.[5]

In the DM-ID, 4 key areas of assessment for paraphilias in persons with intellectual disability were elaborated: cognitive assessment (ie, Ref.[29]), static and dynamic risk assessment,[30,31] phallometric testing,[32] and sociosexual knowledge and attitudes.[32,33] In addition to the typical assessment batteries used for offenders without intellectual disability, because of the issues described earlier, for offenders with intellectual disability an assessment of sexual knowledge and attitudes is especially recommended.[18]

TREATMENT

Before the 1980s there were few programs that provided specialized treatment of persons with intellectual disabilities and those that did were largely based on behavioral suppression paradigms.[9,34] One of the first specialized treatment programs emerged from within the community.[34] Individualized treatment programs were designed based on the needs presented in 6 critical areas (social competency training, sex education, coping skills, responsibility training, relationship training, and treatment to alter deviant sexual arousal). Treatment was provided in the context of natural support networks, and in growth-enhancing but safe environments in natural community settings. Each treatment plan included an active relapse prevention strategy.

Since then there has been several shifts in treatment models. Four differential pathways have been identified as important to matching appropriate treatment to specific offender types.[35] According to this scheme of categorization, avoidant/passive offenders do not actively seek to reoffend but lack appropriate or functional skills or strategies; avoidant/active offenders similarly do not actively seek to reoffend but engage in strategies that are ineffective. In contrast, approach/automatic offenders seek to engage in illegal sex spontaneously and impulsively if the situation is presented. People categorized as approach/explicit offenders actively pursue opportunities to reoffend. Treatment should therefore be tailored to meet the individual needs of each type of offender based in part on their pathway to offense. Some offenders require more focus on habilitative approaches, whereas others require focus on rehabilitative strategies as approaches to self-regulation.[36]

Andrews and Bonta[37] described a 3-part model for consideration in the treatment of all offenders: risk, needs and responsivity. They suggested that the level of service provided should match the relative risk assessed for the individual to reoffend; that treatment should flow from the assessment of the criminogenic needs of the individual that would leave the person vulnerable to reoffense; and that treatment should be provided that is responsive to the needs and strengths of the specific individual, accounting for unique abilities and learning. For persons with intellectual disabilities the evaluation of each of these components of the model requires understanding of the nature of the offense committed and the factors that may reduce recidivism while incorporating the specific learning needs of the individual relative to the disability.

SPECIFIC TREATMENTS
Pharmacologic Treatments

The pharmacologic treatment of paraphilic disorders has recently been reviewed.[38] The article summarizes the English language literature from 1969 to 2009 and concludes with a treatment algorithm consisting of 6 levels of ascending risk and potential harm to the victim. The algorithm begins with psychotherapy (level 1), then adds selective serotonergic reuptake inhibitors for hands-off offenses (level 2), then adds antiandrogens (levels 2–3), then adds or switches to gonadotropin-releasing hormone agonists (GnRH; levels 4–5), and then a combination of all 3 medication types for the most severe (harmful) paraphilias (level 6).

However, the algorithm makes no mention of the special needs of people with intellectual disabilities. The first issue in this group is to accurately diagnose all the sexual and nonsexual problems of the person. As indicated earlier, people with intellectual disabilities have, on average, more problems of both types. The second issue is the importance of obtaining informed consent (described later). The third issue is that people with intellectual disabilities often are already on medications that may interact with new medications. A significant side effect of antiandrogen and GnRH medications is osteoporosis. Many people with intellectual disabilities have osteoporosis because of other risk factors, including anticonvulsant medications, smoking, and physical inactivity. However, osteoporosis can easily be diagnosed by bone densitometry and treated with calcium, vitamin D, and bisphosphonates (even while continuing the medications prescribed to reduce sex drive).

An important issue to remember, and one that is not made clear in the 6-level algorithm described earlier, is that treatments can be tapered once the person has responded to treatment. This fact is often helpful in convincing individuals to try medications to assist them in gaining control of their lives, including their sex lives. The algorithm emphasizes compliance (the difference between level 4 and 5 is primarily one of compliance). GnRH medications are available by intramuscular injection (IM) only and the creators of the algorithm clearly think that IM injections ensure compliance. However, this is only true if there is consent. Some people with intellectual disability are noncompliant not because they do not want to get better but because they are already taking lots of pills or have trouble remembering to take pills. It is important to find out not only whether the person is compliant but also the reason they are thinking of becoming noncompliant. Whichever treatment is agreed on, it is important to reassess the efficacy of the treatment. Including the person in this process is empowering to them and helps to assure them that the treatment has specific goals that are negotiable.

Nonpharmocologic Treatments

Negotiation is a key element in the nonpharmacologic aspects of treatment and these have recently been reviewed.[39] In the case of individuals with intellectual disabilities, it is important to remember that treatment providers have the privilege to serve the person seeking treatment by meeting their needs. People with intellectual disability do not always realize this fact. It is common for workers to think the aim of treatment is to make the workers' lives less stressful. Therefore it is important to show the person with intellectual disability that they are in charge, which can be done by asking them directly whose idea it was to seek treatment and what they personally would like to get out of treatment. Even recalcitrant and reluctant individuals can usually be persuaded that it is worth seeing whether voluntary treatment can improve their lives. It is common for so-called noncompliant people to become enthusiastic participants when the reasons for noncompliance are identified, respected, and addressed. A frequent occurrence is for a man to be referred with "noncompliant" repeated throughout his file. He is noted to never do his written homework assignments and to make excuses to avoid attending group. He seems like a typical unmotivated offender in denial until it is discovered that he is illiterate. Once he is assured he does not need to read or write materials (which he cannot do), the attitude changes. In a similar way, it is common for people with intellectual disabilities to breach curfews, not because they are psychopaths but rather because they do not own a watch, cannot tell time, or are unable to use public transportation.

People with intellectual disabilities are more likely to live in supervised or supported living arrangements, so they are often more closely monitored. Often alterations in living arrangements or routines are more important that medications or therapies. A man who exposes himself to his housemates may be successfully treated by providing him with a housecoat. A man with transvestic interests who steals lingerie may be treated by allowing him to purchase his own lingerie. However, psychotherapy is sometimes also required. At present, there are more than 500 types of psychotherapies. The large number of psychotherapies does not mean that none of them works; to the contrary, it suggests that many different therapies work, some better than others for different individuals. It has been argued that the crucial element in effective therapy is the therapist's belief that the therapy works.[40] Even more effective is when both the therapist and person receiving therapy not only believe in the therapy but also see results.

In the case of individuals with intellectual disabilities it is important to include them in the process. A good way to do this is to introduce them to the idea of a shared series of experiments in which the person receiving therapy tries out suggestions to see whether they work or not. This premise is appealing because it elevates the person from the role of passive patient to that of an active investigator. It also helps minimize the sense of failure when an intervention does not work. It is important to tell the person that the first intervention(s) may not be successful but something can be learned from each change, with the expectation that things will improve. Once this premise is established, the specific therapy is less important than the beliefs of the therapist and client in the possibility of improvement.

Combinations

Pharmacotherapy alone is rarely as effective as a combination of reassurance, recreational and financial support, education, couple's or family therapy (or at least involvement), and psychotherapy. Again, it is best to encourage the person being treated to be involved in choosing which intervention(s) should be pursued, in which combinations and in which order. It is best to deal with the most significant problems first. If the person is homeless, the first effort needs to go into finding shelter. If the person has a life-threatening infection, a trip to emergency room should be the first recommendation. People with intellectual disabilities are often highly adept at prioritizing their needs and their legal and nonharmful wishes should be respected, not only because it is ethical but also because, if they do not agree with the treatment plan, it is unlikely to work.

CHALLENGES TO TREATMENT

Although there are many challenges to treatment, 2 that need to be highlighted are the areas of consent and treatment compliance.

Consent Issues

Ensuring informed consent, whether for treatment or research, can be complicated with persons with intellectual disabilities. Issues such as communication, literacy, and competence are often raised,[41] as well as concerns regarding duress or over-learned compliance to authority.[42] For many individuals it is insufficient to merely ask whether they agree or understand. There is a requirement for due diligence to identify knowledge gaps so that appropriate education is provided. This requirement is especially important in order to obtain true informed consent that is not only given freely but also from accurate information.[43]

Treatment compliance

Persons with intellectual disabilities have been described as highly susceptible to acting in a way that they think will please those in authority.[44] It therefore gives additional value to considering the claim in the sex offender literature that cognitive distortions may be a strategy used by the individual to appease the therapists.[45,46] In order to avoid this problem it is useful to remind the person they are in charge. This statement often surprises not only the person but also their care providers. Take time to explain that all the professionals in the room are employed to assist the person to be as healthy and independent as possible. This assistance includes working toward establishing a fulfilling and legal sexual relationship. Once they are accepted as true, these statements establish a therapeutic relationship that is different from relationships in which the person feels coerced or even punished.

EVALUATION OUTCOME AND LONG TERM RECOMMENDATIONS

With the advent of community living and the closure of institutions for persons with intellectual disabilities, more such persons are residing in the community within their own homes or supported settings. Griffiths[47] noted that there were 2 key aspects to ensuring that treatment integrity is generalized to and maintained long term in the community. The first is that the relative focus on protection and resiliency building must match the level of risk that the individual poses. Individuals posing a higher risk require settings that engage a more active protective focus, including reduction of risk factors, generalization of training to community settings, monitoring skill acquisition of protective factors, and an adherence to ongoing vigilance. Persons who pose lower risks would be provided with a greater focus on resiliency building of proactive skills and active engagement to build self-esteem.

Although both high-risk and low-risk offender groups, as well as those who are in between, need multiple elements in their support plans, and the nature of the setting within the community needs to adapt to match those needs. Iannou and colleagues studied 3 different types of sex offender treatment settings in the community and showed the continuum of services required to meet the needs.[48] The balance of the risks and the rights of individuals in the community requires a shift in focus depending on the needs of the individual. Those individuals posing high risk would have a greater emphasis on risk management, whereas those posing lower risks could reside in residential environments in which rights with regard to community living could take a greater focus. Just as one type of treatment does not suit all offenders, neither does the level of supports needed. Balancing risks and rights is a dynamic process that varies across individuals and over time as treatment success emerges. Regardless of the nature of the setting, the model of building a good life provides a fundamental foundation for long-term therapeutic change.[49]

SUMMARY

People with intellectual disabilities and problematic sexual behaviors have the same rights as those without intellectual disability. Often their needs are more complex. Often they require more support. They are typically more vulnerable. However, fundamentally they are people with the same range of sexual interests and behaviors as the general public. Treatment programs that start with the preceding premises are highly successful.

REFERENCES

1. American Association of Intellectual and Developmental Disability. Definition. Available at: http://www.aaidd.org/intellectual-disability/definition#UKL9r43saA. Accessed October 15, 2013.
2. Hayes S, Shackell P, Mottram P, et al. The prevalence of intellectual disability in a major UK prison. Brit J Learn Disabil 2007;35:162–7.
3. Lindsay WR, Steele L, Smith AH, et al. A community forensic intellectual disability service: twelve year follow-up of referrals, analysis of referral patterns and assessment of harm reduction. Legal Criminol Psych 2006;11:113–30.

4. Nottestad JA, Linaker OM. People with intellectual disabilities sentenced to preventive supervision—mandatory care outside jails and institutions. J Pol Pract Intellect Disabil 2005;2:221–8.

5. Griffiths D. Sexual aggression. In: Gardner W, editor. Aggression and other disruptive behavioral challenges: biomedical and psychosocial assessment and treatment. New York: National Association for Dual Diagnosis; 2002. p. 325–98.

6. Firth S. Psychopathology of sexual abuse in young people with intellectual disability. J Intellect Disabil Res 2001;45:244–52.

7. Brown A, Courtless TF. The mentally retarded offender. In: Allen RC, editor. Readings in law and psychiatry. Baltimore (MA): Johns Hopkins University Press; 1969.

8. Moschella S. The mentally retarded offender: law enforcement and court proceedings. In: Santamour MB, Watson PS, editors. The retarded offender. New York: Praeger Publishing; 1982.

9. Murphy WD, Coleman EM, Haynes MR. Treatment and evaluation issues with the mentally retarded sex offender. In: Greer JD, Stuart IR, editors. The sexual aggressor: current perspectives on treatment. New York: Van Nostrand Reinhold; 1983. p. 21.

10. Santamour MB, West B. The retarded offender and corrections. In: Freidman P, editor. Mental Retardation and the Law. Washington DC: Presidents Committee on Mental Retardation; 1978. p. 25–37.

11. Abel GG, Rouleau J. The nature and extent of sexual assault. In: Marshall WL, Laws DR, Barabarree HE, editors. Handbook of sexual assault. New York: Plenum Press; 1990. p. 9–21.

12. Day K. Male mentally handicapped sex offenders. Br J Psychiatry 1994;165:630–9.

13. Lakin KC, Hill BK, Hauber FA, et al. Changes in age at first admission to residential care for mentally retarded people. Ment Retard 1982;20(5):216–9.

14. Lunsky Y, Frijters J, Griffiths DM, et al. Sexual knowledge and attitudes of men with intellectual disability who sexually offend. J Intellect Dev Disabil 2007;32:74–81.

15. Hingsburger D, Griffiths D, Quinsey V. Detecting counterfeit deviance. Habilitative Mental Healthcare 1991;9:51–4.

16. Hingsburger D. Motives for coprophilia: working with individuals who have been institutionalized with developmental handicaps. J Sex Res 1989;26:139–40.

17. Fletcher R, Loschen E, Stavrakaki C, et al. Diagnostic manual–intellectual disability. Kingston (NY): NADD; 2007.

18. Griffiths D, Fedoroff JP, Richards D, et al. Sexual and gender identify disorders. In: Fletcher R, Loschen E, Stavrakaki C, et al, editors. Diagnostic manual-intellectual disability: a text book of diagnosis of mental disorders in persons with intellectual disabilities. Kingston (NY): NADD Press; 2007. p. 411–57.

19. Eaton L, Menolascino FJ. Psychiatric disorders in the mentally retarded: types, problems, and challenges. Am J Psychiatry 1982;139:1297–303.

20. Reiss S, Levitan G, Szyszko J. Emotional disturbance and mental retardation: diagnostic overshadowing. Habilitative Mental 1982;86:567–74.

21. Fletcher R, Beasley J, Jacobson JW. Supportive services systems for people with dual diagnosis in the USA. In: Bouras N, editor. Psychiatric and behavioural disorders in developmental disabilities and mental retardation. New York: Cambridge University Press; 1999. p. 373–90.

22. Fedoroff JP, Fedoroff BI, Peever C. Consent to treatment issues in sex offenders with developmental delay. In: Griffiths DM, Richards D, Fedoroff P, et al, editors.

Ethical dilemmas: sexuality and developmental disabilities. Kingston (NY): NADD Press; 2002. p. 355–86.

23. Goldberg S. Attachment, parental behaviour, and early development in infants with medical problems. In: Covell K, editor. Readings in child development. Toronto: Neilson; 1995. p. 89–128.

24. McCabe MP. Sexual knowledge, experience and feelings among people with disability. Sex Disabil 1999;17:157–70.

25. Hingsburger D. Erotophobic behavior in people with developmental disabilities. Habilitative Mental Healthcare Newsletter 1992;11:31–4.

26. Sobsey D. Violence and abuse in the lives of people with disabilities. Baltimore (MD): Paul H Brookes Publishing; 1994.

27. Griffiths D, Fedoroff P. Persons with intellectual disabilities who sexually offend. In: Saleh FM, Grudzinskas AJ, Bradford JM, et al, editors. Sex offenders: identification, risk, assessment, treatment, and legal issues. New York: Oxford University Press; 2008. p. 352–74.

28. Day K. Sex offenders with learning disabilities. In: Read SG, editor. Psychiatry in learning disability. London: Sander; 1997. p. 278–306.

29. Broxholme SL, Lindsay W. Development of questionnaire on cognitions related to sex offending. J Intellect Disabil Res 2003;47:472–82.

30. Hanson RK, Harris AJ. Static 2000. Ottawa (Canada): Ottawa, Ontario: Department of Solicitor General; 2000.

31. Hanson RK. The development of a brief actuarial risk scale for sexual offense records. Ottawa (Canada): Department of Solicitor General; 1997.

32. Reye JR, Vollmer TR, Sloman KN, et al. Assessment of deviant arousal in adult male sex offenders with developmental disabilities. J Appl Behav Anal 2006; 39:173–88.

33. McCabe M, Cummins R. The sexual knowledge, experience, feelings and needs of people with mild intellectual disability. Educ Train Ment Retard Dev Disabil 1996;31:13–21.

34. Griffiths D, Quinsey VL, Hingsburger D. Changing sexually inappropriate behaviour. Baltimore (MD): Paul H Brookes Publishing; 1989.

35. Ward T, Hudson SM. A model of the relapse process in sexual offenders. J Interpers Violence 1998;13:700–25.

36. Ward T, Gannon T. Rehabilitation, etiology, and self-regulation: the good lives model of rehabilitation for sexual offenders. Aggress Violent Behav 2006;11: 77–94.

37. Andews DA, Bonta J. The psychology of criminal conduct. 4th edition. Cincinnati (OH): Anderson; 2007.

38. Thibout F, De La Barra F, Gordon H, et al. The World Federation of Societies of Biological Psychiatry (WFSBP) guidelines for the biological treatment of paraphilias. World J Biol Psychiatry 2010;11:604–55.

39. Murphy L, Bradford J, Fedoroff JP. Treatment of paraphilias and paraphilic disorders. In: Gebbard GO, editor. Gebbard's treatments of psychiatric disorders. 5th edition. American Psychiatric Publishing, in press.

40. Frank J, Frank J. Persuasion & healing: a comparative study of psychotherapy. 3rd edition. Baltimore (MD): Johns Hopkins University Press; 1991.

41. Arscott K, Dagnan D, Kroese BS. Assessing the ability of people with a learning disability to give informed consent to treatment. Psychol Med 1999;29:1367–75.

42. Iacono T, Murray V. Issues of informed consent in conducting medical research involving people with intellectual disability. J Appl Res Intellect Disabil 2003;16: 41–51.

43. Dinerstein R, Herr SS, O'Sullivan JL. A guide to consent. Washington, DC: American Association on Mental Retardation; 1999.
44. Flynn MC, Reeves D, Whelan E, et al. The development of a measure for determining the mentally handicapped adult's tolerance of rules and recognition of rights. J Practical Approach 1985;9:18–24.
45. Laws DR. Relapse prevention and sex offenders. New York: Guilford; 1989.
46. Wright RC, Schneider SL. Deviant sexual fantasies as motivated self-deception. In: Schwartz BK, Cellini HR, editors. The sex offender: new insights, treatment innovations and legal developments. Kingston (NJ): Civic Research Institute; 1997. p. 1–14.
47. Griffiths DM. Supporting persons who have sexually offended in the community. European Congress on Mental Health and Intellectual Disability. Estoril, Portugal (Solicited Symposium), September 13, 2013.
48. Iannou S, Griffiths D, Owen F, et al. Managing risk in a culture of rights: Providing support and treatment in community-based settings for persons with intellectual disabilities who sexually offend. ATSA Forum 2014;26(1). Available at: http://newsmanager.commpartners.com/atsa/issues/2014-02-11/4/.html. Accessed January 31, 2014.
49. Ward T, Mann RE, Gannon TA. The good lives model of offender rehabilitation: clinical implications. Aggress Violent Behav 2007;12:87–107.

Treatment and Management of Child Pornography Use

Michael C. Seto, PhD*,
A.G. Ahmed, MBBS, LLM, MSc, MPsychMed, MRCPsych, FRCPC

KEYWORDS

- Child pornography • Pornography • Paraphilias • Treatment • Management
- Sexual self-regulation

KEY POINTS

- Changes in technology, public policy, and law have resulted in a dramatic increase in the number of child pornography offenders presenting for assessment or treatment.
- Not all child pornography use is motivated by pedophilic sexual interests.
- The sex, age, and explicitness of depictions of children are relevant to considering the diagnosis as is the pattern and frequency of child pornography use.
- Child pornography use is sometimes a manifestation of hypersexual or compulsive sexual behavior.
- Comprehensive assessment is essential to effective treatment and risk management of child pornography offenders.
- Treatment and management strategies must take the motivations for child pornography use into account.

INTRODUCTION
Nature of the Problem

With the emergence of Internet technologies and the resulting dramatic increase in availability, affordability, and access to pornography online, there is increasing concern about child pornography use. This concern is predicated on the belief that easy access to child pornography will have undesirable effects, such as the desensitization and normalization of child sexual abuse[1] and future sexual offending against children (for reviews see[2,3]). This concern, in turn, has led to significant public policy changes and new anti–child pornography laws in many jurisdictions. These policy

No disclosures to make.
Royal Ottawa Health Care Group, uOttawa Institute of Mental Health Research, 1145 Carling Avenue, Ottawa, Ontario K1Z 7K4, Canada
* Corresponding author.
E-mail address: michael.seto@theroyal.ca

Psychiatr Clin N Am 37 (2014) 207–214
http://dx.doi.org/10.1016/j.psc.2014.03.004
0193-953X/14/$ – see front matter © 2014 Elsevier Inc. All rights reserved.

psych.theclinics.com

changes and the concomitant investment of law enforcement resources have resulted in a dramatic increase in the number of child pornography users who are entering clinical and forensic settings.[4]

Motivations to Offend and Types of Child Pornography Users

The preferred treatment and management strategy depends on a careful assessment of each user because intervention will depend, in part, on the motivations for child pornography offending and the type of child pornography offender being considered. It will also depend on the risk of reoffending posed by child pornography offenders.[5] Child pornography offender risk assessment is discussed in more detail by Seto.[6]

The first motivation to consider is pedophilia, which is clinically defined as a persistent sexual attraction to prepubescent children.[7] It is intuitive that child pornography use is associated with pedophilia on the assumption that individuals will seek out the kind of pornography they are most interested in. For example, most heterosexual men do not seek out male-male pornography or if they do it is infrequent. Research supports this notion. For example, Seto and colleagues[8,9] found that most (61%) of the 100 child pornography offenders showed greater sexual arousal to depictions of children than adults when assessed in the phallometric laboratory; this was, in fact, a greater proportion than found among sex offenders with child victims, leading to calls for child pornography to be considered a diagnostic indicator of pedophilia.[6,10] Another study in Germany found that most self-identified pedophiles and hebephiles responding to an offer of confidential clinical service admitted to child pornography use.[11] This finding does not mean, however, that child pornography use is synonymous with pedophilia; some child pornography users would not meet the diagnostic criteria for pedophilia, and some pedophiles may not use child pornography.

In some cases, child pornography use might be motivated by hypersexual or compulsive sexual behavior.[12,13] Hypersexual disorder was considered for inclusion in the *Diagnostic and Statistical Manual of Mental Disorders* (Fifth Edition) but was not accepted.[14] In other cases, child pornography use may be a result of reckless or impulsive behavior or accidental access or curiosity. This finding suggests there are different types of child pornography offenders: a paraphilic group comprised of individuals who would meet the diagnosis of pedophilia; a sexually compulsive or hypersexual group who would need assessment and treatment regarding their sexual self-regulation; a group of impulsive, risk-taking individuals who require more general intervention regarding their self-regulation; and a relatively low-need group of accidental or curious users (see[6]).

Assessment and Diagnosis

The assessment and diagnosis of pedophilia (and other paraphilias) is discussed in detail elsewhere in this issue by Seto and colleagues (see also[15]). Self-report is essential to determine the role that hypersexuality or other motivations might play. Because of the stigma associated with the pedophilia label, some child pornography users will claim hypersexuality or nonsexual motivations instead. Differential diagnosis requires careful evaluation of the user's credibility, the legal and other stakes, and relevant behavior. For example, someone who claims hypersexual or compulsive sexual behavior would be expected to show other problematic sexual behavior, such as the use of other forms of illegal or extreme pornography, use of commercial sex services, and online sexual chat. Someone who claimed impulsive or reckless use of child pornography would be unlikely to have organized collections of child pornography (eg, by ethnicity, sex, age, or series of images).

MANAGEMENT GOALS
Sex

Most identified pedophilic individuals are men, and most of the clinical and research literature has focused on male pedophiles.[15] The generalizability of the interventions described later for female pedophiles is unknown. There are sex differences in sexual response and the prevalence of paraphilias, suggesting that paraphilias are less likely to be found in women and that interventions focusing on changing genital sexual arousal patterns may not have the desired subjective sexual arousal effects ([16], though see[17]).

Management versus treatment

Although longitudinal evidence is needed, most clinicians and researchers think paraphilic disorders cannot be cured in the sense that the sexual attraction can be changed; instead, paraphilic disorders need to be managed such that the person no longer experiences distress or impairment. Someone might still have a sexual interest in children, for example, but would not be troubled by their sexual fantasies or urges and would not engage in child pornography use or sexual behavior involving children.

Many clinicians and researchers also think paraphilias can be viewed as similar to sexual orientation with regard to sex; for example, Seto[18] has discussed the evidence that pedophilia, the best understood paraphilia, can be viewed as a sexual orientation with regard to age. This view includes evidence that individuals who admit to having pedophilic interests often report an onset of awareness around the time of puberty or early adolescence, just as most of the population is discovering its interests in males or females or both sexes.

Another consideration in the treatment and management of paraphilias is psychiatric comorbidity (see the article by Seto and colleagues elsewhere in this issue). Some paraphilic individuals will have more than one paraphilia, and paraphilic disorders are often comorbid with mood disorders in particular.[19,20] Effective treatment and management will also need to address these additional conditions. Comorbidity of paraphilias or comorbidity with personality disorder is expected to make effective treatment and management more challenging.

Nonpharmacologic Treatment Options

The psychological treatment of sex offenders, not all of whom would have a paraphilic disorder, is reviewed by Marshall and Marshall in this issue. (Seto, 2008,[15] estimated that approximately 50%–60% of sex offenders with child victims would have pedophilia.) In the following sections, the authors review the literature on the treatment and management of paraphilic disorders, with a special emphasis on pedophilia. The authors also discuss the more limited literature on the treatment and management of child pornography offenders.

Behavioral therapy

One of the earliest evaluated interventions for paraphilic disorders was behavioral therapy, using learning to suppress sexual arousal to paraphilic foci. For example, aversive conditioning techniques were used as early as the 1950s and 1960s for paraphilias, such as fetishism and transvestic fetishism ([21,22]). These aversive conditioning paradigms involved the pairing of sexual arousal to the paraphilic stimulus (eg, photographs of women's shoes) with an aversive stimulus, such as an unpleasant ammonia odor. In a variation called *covert sensitization*, the aversive stimulus is imagined, for example, imagining being discovered by one's spouse or family members while engaging in paraphilic behavior.

There is evidence that individuals can learn greater voluntary control over their sexual arousal through behavioral conditioning [23,24]. However, it is unclear how long the effects last; much depends on the individual's willingness to use that voluntary control in an otherwise sexually arousing situation (eg, being near a paraphilic stimulus, such as child pornography or being in the presence of a prepubescent child). Research showing that pretreatment assessments of sexual arousal are stronger predictors of reoffending than posttreatment assessments suggests the effects of treatment on sexual responding likely fade over time, requiring periodic monitoring and booster sessions as needed.[25]

Some therapists have attempted to positively reinforce greater sexual arousal to normative cues (to adults, in the case of pedophiles); but there is very limited evidence that one can condition greater sexual arousal to an initially nonpreferred stimulus (for a review, see[26]). Moreover, the effects of positive conditioning to increase sexual arousal to previously nonpreferred categories are small in magnitude.

Self-management Strategies

The most common forms of psychosocial therapies for dealing with paraphilic disorders that result in criminal involvement involve cognitive-behavioral techniques within a relapse-prevention or self-regulation framework[27] (see,[28] also discussed elsewhere in this issue). The relapse prevention framework was adapted from the addictions field, based on some of the similarities between apparently compulsive sexual behavior and compulsive substance use. The self-regulation framework is built on relapse-prevention principles but recognizes that some individuals are not motivated to refrain from the problematic behavior; instead, they seek out opportunities to offend. Thus, the self-regulation framework distinguishes between approach and avoidance pathways to sexual offending.

Both relapse-prevention and self-regulation treatments involve a functional analysis of paraphilic behavior in order to identify the antecedents, chains of thoughts, and behaviors that lead up to acting on paraphilic interests. The therapist and client then use that functional analysis to identify risky situations and triggers. For example, many paraphilic individuals might feel less able to manage their paraphilic fantasies or urges when they have a low mood, are under stress, or experience some kind of serious interpersonal conflict. Then, with this knowledge of risky situations and triggers, therapy aims to help the client develop individual coping strategies.

The principles from the Good Lives Model are also frequently included.[27] This relatively new sex offender treatment model posits the importance of positive life goals and takes a more holistic and strengths-based approach than traditional sex offender treatment, as part of the positive psychology movement in recent years. The Good Lives Model recognizes that the paraphilic interest can be a major part of someone's life and fulfills various needs (eg, not only sexual gratification but also mood regulation, socially, and so forth). If that paraphilic interest is effectively managed, then what will fill the void that has been created? The Good Lives Model suggests that individuals who successfully inculcate prosocial life goals and build on their strengths will be less likely to reoffend. The Good Lives Model also recognizes that sexual offending fulfills needs that need be fulfilled by prosocial behaviors and goals.

The Internet Sex Offender Treatment Program (i-SOTP) was developed and is now implemented as the national program for child pornography offenders on probation in the United Kingdom.[29] The i-SOTP draws on concepts and content from relapse prevention, the Good Lives Model, and other contemporary sex offender treatment approaches. Designed to be less intense than the national program for contact sex offenders, the i-SOTP involves 20 to 30 sessions, usually in a group format, for child pornography offenders with no history of contact sexual offenses. These sessions are organized into 6 modules: (1) motivation to change, (2) functional analysis of online offending behavior, (3) attitudes and beliefs, (4) interpersonal deficits, (5) self-regulation skills, and (6) relapse-prevention skills and setting new life goals. A notable feature of this program is the importance given at the beginning of the program in addressing motivation to change. A pre-post treatment evaluation showed significant changes on self-report measures of treatment targets, but the analysis did not address treatment attrition and did not include a suitable comparison group.

Another nonexclusive option involves self-help content influenced by relapse-prevention and addiction approaches available online at croga.org. This site was originally developed to provide anonymous self-help for individuals concerned about their online behavior and is now maintained by the Lucy Faithfull Foundation in the United Kingdom.

Pharmacologic Treatment Options

The pharmacologic treatment of paraphilias is covered by Thibaut and Bradford in this issue.

Evaluation of Outcome, Adjustment of Treatment, and Long-term Recommendations

Relapse is common for pedophilic sex offenders with child victims without effective management of pedophilia. The longest-term follow-up studies of pedophilic sex offenders currently available have found that approximately 30% to 40% were identified as committing a new sexual offense after up to 30 years of opportunity to offend.[30,31] Some of the remaining cases might also have committed new sexual offenses without getting caught, as recidivism data are almost always obtained by accessing data on criminal charges or convictions. Besides underestimating new offending, new charges or convictions for sexual offenses are blunt outcome measures because they do not necessarily capture the severity of any new offenses or capture the clinical distress or impairment as a result of continuing paraphilic fantasies, urges, and arousal.

In contrast to these long-term findings for pedophilic sex offenders with child victims, the emerging evidence on child pornography offenders suggests they are relatively low risk to reoffend in the first few years of opportunity, especially if they have no prior criminal history and no history of contact sexual offending.[32,33] These results suggest that pedophilic disorder, which is expected among the majority of child pornography users, is not a necessary or sufficient cause of sexual offending in the future; variation in antisocial tendencies is critical, with more antisocial child pornography offenders being more likely to sexually offend.[6]

As is true for the sex offender field more generally, long-term, well-controlled treatment evaluations are needed and have been frequently called for in reviews of the literature. The results of randomized clinical trials are particularly important. Ethical and scientific objections to the use of randomized clinical trials in sex offender treatment evaluation have been addressed.[28,34] At a minimum, the field needs outcome evaluations involving wait-list controls and/or assignment to alternative treatment conditions.

SUMMARY

The treatment and management of child pornography use depends on the motivation for child pornography offending. Individuals who genuinely accessed child pornography out of curiosity or as part of nonsexual thrill seeking are unlikely to have a paraphilic disorder. However, many individuals will claim accidental access or curiosity as a motivation, and the credibility of these explanations requires a comprehensive sexological assessment.

Individuals who access child pornography as part of a pattern of hypersexual or compulsive behavior share treatment needs with those who access child pornography because it reflects their sexual interest in children. Namely, both groups of individuals are likely to require treatment emphasizing increased self-regulation skills in the sexual domain delivered in the form of cognitive-behavioral therapy and possibly with the aid of sex drive–reducing medications. Sexual self-regulation deficits are the one domain where child pornography offenders have been found to score higher than contact sex offenders.[35]

The World Federation of Societies of Biological Psychiatry suggests an algorithm based on the intensity of paraphilic disorder and severity of consequences if the paraphilic disorder is not effectively managed (eg, pedophilia and sexual offenses against children, arousal to sexual violence or nonconsensual suffering and rape).[36] Given the serious side effects and quality-of-life impacts of antiandrogen or Gonadotropin releasing hormone (GnRH) agonist treatment, this medication should be reserved for cases whereby other options have not worked or the risk of serious harm is high.

Pedophilic individuals may also require behavioral conditioning to increase voluntary control over sexual arousal to children. Some pedophilic individuals might require little to no intervention because they have a low sex drive and/or high self-regulation.[37] Nonetheless, such individuals might experience distress or some impairment in functioning and may require supportive psychotherapy.

PREVENTION

A challenge in the treatment and management of paraphilic individuals is reaching them before serious negative consequences have already occurred. Paraphilias are stigmatized, making it less likely for individuals to seek help, especially from general practitioners and nonspecialists. In particular, pedophilia is highly stigmatized. An interesting secondary prevention model has been developed in Germany to address this problem.[38] The Dunkelfeld Project used foundation funding to advertise clinical assessment and treatment services for individuals who were concerned about their sexual interest in children. To date, several hundred individuals have been treated; evaluation efforts are ongoing (dont-offend.org). In the United States, Stop It Now (stopitnow.org) provides a confidential hotline with resources and a referral directory for individuals who are concerned about their sexual interests in children or in sexually assaulting adults.

FUTURE DIRECTIONS

Research is beginning to emerge on the assessment, diagnosis, and treatment of online child pornography offenders.[6] There is an urgent need for a better understanding of the different trajectories individuals might follow to child pornography use, beginning with broad distinctions between paraphilic motivations (such as pedophilia or hebephilia), hypersexuality, and less overtly sexual motivations, such as thrill seeking or curiosity. The risk to offend again and, thus, treatment and management needs are likely to differ across these different types of child pornography offenders. More broadly, there is literature to draw on in developing and evaluating treatment approaches for child pornography offenders, particularly the literature on the treatment of paraphilias and treatment of sex offenders. In all of these areas, however, more methodologically rigorous evaluations are needed to determine the best way forward.

REFERENCES

1. Lanning K. Child molesters: A behavioral analysis. National Center for Missing and Exploited Children 2001. Available at: www.missingkids.com/en_US/publications/NC70.pdf. Accessed March 24, 2014.
2. Malamuth NM, Addison T, Koss M. Pornography and sexual aggression: Are there reliable effects and can we understand them? Annual Review of Sex Research 2000;11:26–91.
3. Marshall WL. Revisiting the use of pornography by sexual offenders: Implications for theory and practice. Journal of Sexual Aggression 2000;6:67–77.
4. United States Sentencing Commission. Report to the congress: federal child pornography offenses. 2012. Available at: http://www.ussc.gov/Legislative_and_Public_Affairs/Congressional_Testimony_and_Reports/Sex_Offense_Topics/201212_Federal_Child_Pornography_Offenses. Accessed November 1, 2013.
5. Reid JA, Beauregard E, Fedina KM, et al. Employing mixed methods to explore motivational patterns of repeat sex offenders. J Crim Justice 2013. http://dx.doi.org/10.1016/j.jcrimjus.2013.06.008.
6. Seto MC. Internet sex offenders. Washington, DC: American Psychological Association; 2013.
7. American Psychiatric Association. Diagnostic and statistical manual of mental disorders. 5th edition. Washington, DC: Author; 2013.
8. Seto MC, Cantor JM, Blanchard R. Child pornography offenses are a valid diagnostic indicator of pedophilia. J Abnorm Psychol 2006;115:610–5.
9. Seto MC, Hanson RK, Babchishin KM. Contact sexual offending by men with online sexual offenses. Sex Abuse 2011;23:124–45.
10. Seto MC. Child pornography use and Internet solicitation in the diagnosis of pedophilia. Arch Sex Behav 2010;39:591–3. http://dx.doi.org/10.1007/s10508-010-9603-6.
11. Neutze J, Seto MC, Schaefer GA, et al. Predictors of child pornography offenses and child sexual abuse in a community sample of pedophiles and hebephiles. Sex Abuse 2011;23:212–42.
12. Delmonico DL, Griffin EJ. Ilegal images: Critical issues and strategies for addressing child pornography use. Holyoke, MA: NEARI Press; 2013.
13. Seto MC, Reeves L, Jung S. Motives for child pornography offending: the explanations given by the offenders. Journal of Sexual Aggression 2010;16:169–80.
14. Kafka MP. Hypersexual disorder: a proposed diagnosis for DSM-V. Arch Sex Behav 2010;39:377–400.
15. Seto MC. Pedophilia and sexual offending against children: theory, assessment, and intervention. Washington, DC: American Psychological Association; 2008.
16. Chivers ML, Seto MC, Lalumière ML, et al. Agreement of self-reported and genital measures of sexual arousal among men and women: A meta-analysis. Arch Sex Behav 2010;39:5–56.
17. Chivers ML, Roy C, Grimbos T, et al. Specificity of sexual arousal for sexual activities in men and women with conventional and masochistic sexual interests [online first]. Arch Sex Behav 2013. [Epub ahead of print].
18. Seto MC. Is pedophilia a sexual orientation? Arch Sex Behav 2012;41:231–6.
19. Freund K, Seto MC, Kuban M. Frotteurism and the theory of courtship disorder. In: Laws DR, O'Donohue WT, editors. Sexual deviance: Theory, assessment and treatment. New York: Guildford; 1997. p. 111–30.
20. Kafka MP, Hennen J. A DSM-IV axis I comorbidity study of males (n = 120) with paraphilias and paraphilia-related disorders. Sex Abuse 2002;14:349–66.

21. Marks IM, Gelder MG. Transvestism and fetishism: clinical and psychological changes during faradic aversion. Br J Psychiatry 1967;113:711–30.
22. Raymond M. Case of fetishism treated by aversion therapy. Br Med J 1956;2: 854–6.
23. Lalumière ML, Earls CM. Voluntary control of penile responses as a function of stimulus duration and instructions. Behav Assess 1992;14:121–32.
24. Mahoney JM, Strassberg DS. Voluntary control of male sexual arousal. Arch Sex Behav 1991;20:1–16.
25. Rice ME, Quinsey VL, Harris GT. Sexual recidivism among child molesters released from a maximum security psychiatric institution. J Consult Clin Psychol 1991;59:381–6.
26. Hoffmann H. The role of classical conditioning in sexual arousal. In: Janssen E, editor. The psychophysiology of sex. Bloomington, IN: University of Indiana Press; 2007. p. 261–77.
27. McGrath R, Cumming G, Burchard B, et al. Current practices and emerging trends in sexual abuser management: the safer society 2009 North American survey. Brandon (VT): Safer Society Press; 2010.
28. Marshall WL, Marshall LE. The utility of the random controlled trial for evaluating sexual offender treatment: the gold standard or an inappropriate strategy? Sex Abuse 2007;19:175–91.
29. Middleton D, Mandeville-Norden R, Hayes E. Does treatment work with Internet sex offenders? Emerging findings from the Internet Sex Offender Treatment Programme (i-SOTP). Journal of Sexual Aggression 2009;15:5–19.
30. Hanson RK, Steffy RA, Gauthier R. Long-term recidivism of child molesters. J Consult Clin Psychol 1993;61:646–52.
31. Prentky RA, Knight RA, Lee AF. Risk factors associated with recidivism among extrafamilial child molesters. J Consult Clin Psychol 1997;65:141–9.
32. Eke AW, Seto MC. Risk assessment of online offenders for law enforcement. In: Ribisl K, Quayle E, editors. Internet child pornography: understanding and preventing on-line child abuse. Devon (United Kingdom): Willan; 2012. p. 148–68.
33. Eke AW, Seto MC, Williams J. Examining the criminal history and future offending of child pornography offenders: an extended prospective follow-up study. Law Hum Behav 2011;35:466–78.
34. Seto MC, Marques JK, Harris GT, et al. Good science and progress in sex offender treatment are intertwined: a response to Marshall and Marshall (2007). Sex Abuse 2008;20:247–55.
35. Webb L, Craissati J, Keen S. Characteristics of Internet child pornography offenders: a comparison with child molesters. Sex Abuse 2007;19:449–65.
36. Thibaut F, Barra FD, Gordon H, et al, WFSBP Task Force. The World Federation of Societies of Biological Psychiatry (WFSBP) guidelines for the biological treatment of paraphilias. World J Biol Psychiatry 2010;11:604–55.
37. Babchishin KM, Hanson RK, VanZuylen H. Online child pornography offenders are different: A meta-analysis of the characteristics of online and offline sex offenders against children [online first]. Arch Sex Behav 2014. [Epub ahead of print].
38. Beier KM, Neutze J, Mundt IA, et al. Encouraging self-identified pedophiles and hebephiles to seek professional help: first results of the Prevention Project Dunkelfeld (PPD). Child Abuse Negl 2009;33:545–9.

Sexual Sadism in Sexual Offenders and Sexually Motivated Homicide

Peer Briken, MD, FECSM[a],*, Dominique Bourget, MD, FRCPC[b], Mathieu Dufour, MD, FRCPC[b]

KEYWORDS

- Sexual sadism • Paraphilic disorder • Sexual homicide • Diagnosis • Assessment
- Treatment

KEY POINTS

- Distinguish sexual sadism disorder from consensual bondage & discipline, dominance & submission, sadism & masochism (BDSM) practices.
- The categorical diagnosis of sexual sadism has weaknesses in reliability and validity.
- In the forensic context, dimensionally and behaviorally oriented assessment procedures are helpful.
- Sexual sadism increases the risk for reoffending in sexual offenders.
- Therapy for sexual sadistic offenders is a specific challenge with particular treatment goals and treatment approaches.

NATURE OF THE PROBLEM

Problems have been identified surrounding the definition, operationalization, and assessment of sexual sadism that have clouded our understanding of it. There is a wide range of normal sexual expressions, and there are only normative criteria for a distinction between healthy and nonhealthy forms of sexual behavior; this can lead to confusion between (1) variants of behavior, (2) problematic or deviant behaviors, and (3) disorders.

BDSM (bondage & discipline, dominance & submission, sadism & masochism) is characterized by consensual sexual preferences and activities. Criticism of BDSM

Disclosure: P. Briken is consultant for Dr Pfleger GmbH (Bamberg, Germany). The remaining authors have nothing to disclose.
[a] Institute for Sex Research & Forensic Psychiatry, University Medical Centre Hamburg-Eppendorf, University of Hamburg, Martinistrasse 52, Hamburg D-20246, Germany; [b] Forensic Program, Department of Psychiatry, The Royal Ottawa Hospital, University of Ottawa, 1145 Carling Avenue, Ottawa, Ontario K1Z 7K4, Canada
* Corresponding author.
E-mail address: briken@uke.uni-hamburg.de

0193-953X/14/$ – see front matter © 2014 Elsevier Inc. All rights reserved.

Abbreviations	
BDSM	Bondage & discipline, dominance & submission, sadism & masochism
DSM	*Diagnostic and Statistical Manual of Mental Disorders*
ICD	International Classification of Diseases
MSI	Multiphasic Sex Inventory
PPG	Penile plethysmography
SES	Sexual Experiences Survey
SORAG	Sex Offender Risk Appraisal Guide
SSSS	Severe Sexual Sadism Scale

activists, and of scientists, is accompanied by the demand to remove the criteria of sexual sadism from the diagnostic systems and accept BDSM as sexual practice.[1] In a representative Australian study, 1.8% of sexually active individuals (2.2% men, 1.3% women) were engaged in BDSM practices in the previous year.[2] BDSM practitioners did not reveal increased dissatisfaction, anxiety, or sexual problems. In a study by Connolly,[3] no differences between BDSM practitioners and the test norms of 7 psychometric tests for the assessment of mental disorder was found. Therefore, it is extremely important to differentiate sexual sadism as a disorder from the pathologizing and stigmatization of BDSM practices. However, some men and, more rarely, women consult professionals because their sexual sadistic interests or practices cause distress and/or impairment, that is, by leading to conflicts between fantasies, behaviors, and values of the individual.

Clinically more important is the relationship between sexual sadism disorder and sexual offending, especially the relevance for very violent forms such as sexual homicide. Sexual homicide is a very rare and peculiar offense with some characteristics that differ from other forms of violent or sexual crime. This specific offense confronts relatives, perpetrators, and experts with the finiteness of life and thereby with existential questions. Above all there is no direct witness to report the offense, so knowledge is limited to what perpetrators say and what one can evaluate from the crime scene. Despite its scarcity, sexual homicide, especially against children, is the crime that causes the vast bulk of negative reporting about sexual offenders in the lay press. Thereby, despite its relative rareness, it may correlate with the extremely negative perception of sexual offending in general and child sexual abuse more specifically. Other characteristics of sexual homicide correspond to sexual or violent offending in general. Sexual sadism in relation to sexual homicide has been discussed since the early descriptions of von Krafft-Ebing[4] or those of the "typical" sadistic (sexual) murderer by Brittain[5] as a weird, emotionally detached, isolated person. Rare but extreme and very severe forms of disturbed behaviors often illuminate the less severe forms. At the same time, there seems to be some kind of mystification of the most awful incidents and perpetrators that may lead to emotional, subjective, and less scientific views concerning the problem.

The aim of this article is to give a clinically oriented narrative overview about the forensically relevant forms of sexual sadism disorder and its relationship to a specific type of offense: sexual homicide.

DEFINITION
Sexual Sadism

In the International Statistical Classification of Diseases and Related Health Problems (ICD-10[6]), sexual sadism is conceptualized as a paraphilia with "a preference for sexual activities involving the infliction of pain or humiliation, or bondage." In the *Diagnostic and Statistical Manual of Mental Disorders* (5th edition) (DSM-5), revisions were made to differentiate between the behavior itself and the disorder arising from that behavior, helping to distinguish between unusual sexual interests and mental disorders involving these desires or behaviors. In DSM-5, sexual sadism disorder is defined as "recurrent and intense sexual arousal from the physical or psychological suffering of another person, as manifested by fantasies, urges, or behaviors."[7]

Symptom criteria in DSM-5

DSM-5 criteria for sexual sadism disorder are as follows:

A. Over a period of at least 6 months, recurrent and intense sexual arousal from the physical or psychological suffering of another person, as manifested by fantasies, urges, or behaviors.
B. The individual has acted on these sexual urges with a nonconsenting person, or the sexual urges and fantasies cause clinically significant distress or impairment in social, occupational, or other important areas of functioning.

The DSM provides 2 distinct specifiers: "In a controlled environment" where opportunities to engage in the behaviors are restricted, and "In full remission" when criterion B has not been met for at least 5 years in an uncontrolled environment.

Table 1 is illustrative of the evolution of symptom criteria for sexual sadism over the past 25 years.

Sexual Homicide

Many studies used Ressler and colleagues'[11] description for a defined criteria list for inclusion in their studies on sexual homicide. For this definition, at least 1 of the criteria in **Box 1** has to be fulfilled.

Table 1		
Evolution of DSM criteria for sexual sadism		
Criteria from DSM-IIIR[8]	**Criteria from DSM-IV[9]**	**Criteria from DSM-IV-TR[10]**
A. Over a period of at least 6 mo, recurrent intense sexual urges and sexually arousing fantasies involving acts (real, not simulated) in which the psychological or physical suffering (including humiliation) of the victim is sexually exciting to the person	A. Over a period of at least 6 mo, recurrent, intense sexually arousing fantasies, sexual urges, or behaviors involving acts (real, not simulated) in which the psychological or physical suffering (including humiliation) of the victim is sexually exciting to the person	A. Over a period of at least 6 mo, recurrent, intense sexually arousing fantasies, sexual urges, or behaviors involving acts (real, not simulated) in which the psychological or physical suffering (including humiliation) of the victim is sexually exciting to the person
B. The person has acted on these urges, or is markedly distressed by them	B. The fantasies, sexual urges, or behaviors cause clinically significant distress or impairment in social, occupational, or other important areas of functioning	B. The person has acted on these urges with a nonconsenting person, or the sexual urges or behaviors cause marked distress or interpersonal difficulty

Abbreviations: DSM, *Diagnostic and Statistical Manual of Mental Disorders*; IIIR, 3rd edition, revision; IV, 4th edition; IV-TR, 4th edition, text revision.

> **Box 1**
> **Criteria list to define sexual homicide**
>
> - Attempted or completed sexual intercourse (oral, anal, or vaginal)
> - Exposure of the primary or secondary sexual parts of the victim's body
> - Victim's being left naked or seminaked
> - Sexual positioning of the victim's body
> - Insertion of foreign objects into the victim's body cavities
> - Semen on or near the victim's body
> - Substitute sexual activity (eg, masturbation, exhibitionistic or voyeuristic behavior)
> - Sexual interest admitted to by the offender
> - Sadistic fantasies admitted to by the offender
>
> *Data from* Ressler RK, Burgess AW, Douglas JE. Sexual homicide: patterns and motives. Lexington (MA): Lexington Books; 1988.

In a recently published article, Sewall and colleagues[12(p83)] used the following broader definition: sexual homicide "refers to those homicides in which sexual activity (including masturbation) occurs with the victim present before, during, or after death."

CLINICAL FINDINGS
Physical Examination

Besides a general physical examination, in certain cases further somatic findings should be used within the diagnostic process (eg, sex hormones, neuroimaging, chromosome analysis, examination of genitals). A standardized assessment includes a sex hormone profile to screen for abnormal hormone levels. Such a profile usually consists of free and total testosterone, follicle-stimulating hormone, luteinizing hormone, estradiol, prolactin, and progesterone.[13] If possible, an inspection and, in suspect cases, a urological examination of the genitals may be useful. Rettenberger and colleagues[14] found a rate of nearly 18% with genital abnormalities in sexual homicide perpetrators (ie, phimosis, cryptorchidism).

There is evidence of biological abnormalities associated with sexual sadism in sex offenders. Gratzer and Bradford[15] compared offender and offense characteristics of 29 sexually sadistic criminals with a control group of 28 men who had committed nonsadistic criminal sex offences. These groups were then compared with a previously published descriptive study of a sample of 30 men who were diagnosed with sexual sadism.[16] Gratzer and Bradford[15] found that more than half (55%) of the sadists had neurological findings indicating temporal lobe abnormalities. There is support for the role of temporal-limbic neural pathways in sexual arousal[17] and aggression.[18] Briken and colleagues[19] analyzed psychiatric court reports of 166 sexual homicide perpetrators and found a rate of 30% with notable signs of brain abnormalities. In the group of sexual homicide perpetrators with such signs, sexual sadism was diagnosed in 50% of the men (vs 31% of the others). In another study with the same sample,[20] the same group investigated the prevalence of the chromosome abnormality XYY, and found a higher rate of XYY chromosome abnormality in the sexual homicide perpetrators (1.8%) than in the general population (0.01%).

Rating scales (**Table 2**) can complement the clinical diagnosis of sexual sadism. Other risk assessment procedures such as the Static-99,[21] the Stable 2007,[22] and the SVR-20[23] can also be useful.

Table 2 Rating scales in the assessment of sexual sadism	
Severe Sexual Sadism Scale (SSSS)	The SSSS[24–26] is a file-based observer rating of pertinent crime-scene behaviors used as a screening tool for the assessment of sexual sadism in forensic cases. The scale consists of 11 dichotomous (yes/no) items that code behavioral indicators of severe sexual sadism within sexual offenses. Reliability and criterion validity for the clinical diagnosis of sexual sadism were reported to be good[27]
The Multiphasic Sex Inventory (MSI)	The MSI[28] is a 300-item, true-false, self-report questionnaire consisting of statements about sexual activities, problems, and experiences. It is primarily intended to be used in assessing sexual offenders to develop treatment plans and to assess progress during treatment. The MSI has 20 scales that include a variety of measures for sexual deviance
Kurt Freund Paraphilia Scales	Kurt Freund developed a series of scales for the standardized diagnostic procedure and assessment of paraphilic interests, which are freely available on the Internet (http://individual.utoronto.ca/ray_blanchard/index_files/EPES.html)[29]
Sex Offender Risk Appraisal Guide (SORAG)	The SORAG was developed[30] as a modification of the Violence Risk Appraisal Guide.[31] Items that predict violent recidivism by sexual offenders were added or revised. Fourteen items assess child and adolescent adjustment, criminal history, psychopathy, and atypical sexual interests: living with both biological parents until age 16, elementary school maladjustment, history of alcohol problems, marital history, nonviolent offense history, victim sex/age, failure on prior conditional release, age at index offense, meeting DSM criteria for any personality disorder and for schizophrenia, phallometrically measured atypical sexual arousal, and Psychopathy Checklist-Revised score.[32] Several studies have supported the predictive validity of the SORAG for sexual and violent recidivism (eg, Refs.[33,34])
Sexual Experiences Survey (SES)	The SES[35] is a 17-item dichotomous (yes/no) scale in which individuals are asked if they have ever had sexual contact with someone who did not want it, ranging from argument to intercourse involving physical force. The SES has been validated in studies of sexual coercion and rape in community samples[36,37]

Diagnostic Modalities

Important issues in taking a sexual history among sexual sadistic patients and sexual homicide perpetrators are:

- Development and content of sexual fantasies: age of onset, frequency and masturbation practice, sexual fantasies in childhood, adolescence, and adulthood
- Detailed exploration of various sadistic and other paraphilic (ie, voyeuristic, fetishistic, transvestistic, pedophilic) interests or activities
- Fantasies, desires, impulses, and behavior within and beyond the partnership
- Pornography consumption (including the use of sadistic and/or violent pornography)
- Sadistic activities with prostitutes
- Experience of sexual and/or other violent assaults in childhood, adolescence or adulthood (as victim or witness)
- Sexual and general delinquency-criminal prosecutions

As diagnostic tools in addition to the DSM and the ICD, penile plethysmography (PPG) and indicators of crime scene behavior have been used. **Table 3** presents a description of common diagnostic tools.

Imaging

Little is known about the neural mechanisms associated with sexual sadism. Early studies using computed tomography scans revealed that sadistic offenders (41%) were more likely than 2 groups of nonsadists (11% and 13%) to have right-sided temporal horn abnormalities.[41,42] To the authors' knowledge there are no studies investigating sexual homicide perpetrators systematically with modern imaging techniques. Preliminary findings of recent research using functional magnetic resonance imaging to investigate the neural mechanisms underlying pain observation in sadists suggest that sadists may have a heightened sensitivity to pain in comparison with nonsadistic sexual offenders.[43] In this study, 15 violent male sexual offenders were assigned to sadist (n = 8) and nonsadist (n = 7) groups based on scores from the SSSS.[26] In response to pictures depicting a person in pain, sadistic offenders exhibited increased activity in the left amygdala, and rated the pain pictures higher on pain severity than nonsadistic offenders. There was a positive association between pain severity ratings and activity in the left anterior insula in sadists that was not present in nonsadists. Sadists also showed greater connectivity between the left amygdala and right anterior insula during pain observation, and demonstrated increased activity in the right temporoparietal junction when viewing both pain and no-pain pictures. Harenski and colleagues[43] suggested that the study findings may reflect context-dependent activation of brain regions in sexual sadists that differs across group, as opposed to structural abnormalities within these brain regions.

Pathology

Epidemiology of sexual sadism disorder and sexual homicide

The categorical diagnosis of sexual sadism disorder has raised considerable controversy over its reliability and validity (eg, Refs.[30,44,45]). This fact, in combination with the extreme differences of the samples studied, is the reason why the prevalence of sexual sadism disorder varies widely and is almost exclusively investigated in sex offenders. Krueger[46] reported a prevalence from 2% to 30% for forensic samples. In a representative sample of incarcerated sexual offenders from Austria, Eher and colleagues[47] found a DSM-IV-TR[10] diagnosis of sexual sadism in 6% (most prominent in rapists with a prevalence near 10%). In a recent study by Mokros and colleagues,[48] taxometric analyses based on the SSSS showed that the underlying structure of forensic sexual sadism may fit better into a dimensional and not into a categorical construct.

Because of the variable definitions used, differing methods of obtaining data, and transcultural impact, the rate of sexual homicide ranges from 3% to 22% of all homicides.[12] The prevalence of sexual sadism (using DSM-IV criteria) in a large sample of sexual homicide perpetrators was 37%.[49]

Course

Remarkable or inappropriate sexual behavior in children and adolescents sometimes leads to child and adolescent psychiatric evaluations. However, sexual sadistic behavior in this context is extremely rare. In clinical reports, investigators describe early imprinting sexual experiences, especially sexual combined with physical traumatizations, extreme oversexualization, and overstimulation by primary caregivers or, on the other side, sexual scruples in relationships to caregivers. The theory that paraphilic

Table 3
Comparison of diagnostic tools

DSM, ICD	The DSM and the ICD have been widely used as categorical diagnostic tools in the assessment of sexual sadism despite criticism over methodological issues. Reliance on self-reports is a limitation in the forensic context
Phallometric assessment (penile plethysmography; PPG)	PPG measures sexual arousal by monitoring changes in penile tumescence while the individual is presented with auditory and (or) visual stimuli that describe or depict sexual interactions involving different partners and types of behavior. The sexual events are designed to vary with respect to age, gender, degree of consent, coercion, and violence portrayed (sexual and nonsexual)[13]
	PPG studies have not consistently identified sexually sadistic rapists and nonsexually sadistic rapists based on their sexual arousal to nonsexual violence. Healey and colleagues[38] suggested that these inconsistent findings might actually reflect the poor validity of the DSM, as sexual sadists are usually identified using DSM diagnostic criteria to which PPG data are compared
	Sexual arousal to violence and injury may distinguish sexual sadists from nonsadists.[39] Seto and colleagues[39] used phallometric measures to test sexual sadism as an explanation of rapists' arousal pattern, with a nonforensic sample of 3 groups of men recruited from the community: 18 self-identified sadists, 22 with some sadistic interests who did not meet all of the study's sadist criteria, and 23 nonsadists. Sadists had significantly greater subjective and genital responses to stories involving violence and injury in comparison with stories not involving violence and injury. This result was not seen with stimuli involving nonconsent compared with those involving consent
Crime-scene behaviors	In attempts to improve agreement across diagnosticians, several studies have focused on the use of indicators of crime-scene behaviors of convicted sex offenders to measure sexual sadism. The criminal behavior of sexual sadists has been described as highly planned and structured, compulsive, ritualized, and violent, and includes torture, mutilation, and humiliation or degradation of the victim (eg, Refs.[16,40])
	Kingston and colleagues[30] used the SORAG to control for level of risk in an examination of the predictive validity of various sexual sadism indicators: a DSM diagnosis of sexual sadism, severity of sexual violence, level of nonsexual violence during the offense, and PPG scores indicating sexual arousal to violence (sexual and nonsexual). Study participants were 586 adult men convicted of a sexual offense and assessed in a sexology clinic. The SORAG best predicted violent recidivism, whereas a DSM diagnosis of sexual sadism was unrelated to recidivism. SORAG scores and PPG scores both significantly predicted sexual recidivism of offenders
	Crime-scene indicators may distinguish between characteristics of sexual sadism and sexual homicide.[38] Healey and colleagues[38] investigated 268 male offenders (182 sexual aggressors of women and 86 sexual murderers) incarcerated in a Canadian penitentiary, and found that only 40% of crime-scene indicators for sexual sadism (ie, premeditation, the use of physical restraints, mutilation, and humiliation) were significantly related to a clinical diagnosis of sexual sadism based on DSM-III-R criteria.[8] As humiliation and mutilation were significantly associated with a diagnosis of sexual sadism and with sexual homicide, Healey and colleagues[38] suggested that 2 distinct types of sexually sadistic offenders (those who murder and those who do not) may exist and be distinguished by whether they humiliate or mutilate their victims

sexual behaviors in adults represent a "reversal of a defeat in childhood"[50] has been offered as one explanation.[51,52] Over time the symptoms may show progression.

Because age is one of the main variables affecting sexual drive, and because there is a decline in sexual desire and activity in middle-aged and elderly individuals compared with adolescents or young adults, sexual sadistic interests may lose some of their dynamics (in the sense of biological drive) across the life span. In a sample of sexual homicide in Germany,[53] perpetrators' recidivism with any violent reoffence was associated with age-related factors (younger age at first sexual offense, at the sexual homicide, and at time of release, and duration of detention). However, even with decreased biological drive the individual's sexual interest or preference does not change automatically.

Typologies of sexual homicide perpetrators

Many attempts have been made to typologize sexual homicide perpetrators. Some typologies use the victim type or the number of victims as a criterion to distinguish these offenders:

- Women versus men (or with a homosexual background)
- Children/adolescents versus adults
- Much older victims versus victims of the same age range
- Serial (eg, $\geq$2–3 homicides as separate events) versus single victim

Other typologies analyze a combination of crime-scene analysis, previous criminal and psychiatric history, and psychological aspects. One of the most influential typologies was the organized/disorganized typology proposed by Ressler and colleagues.[11] The organized offender type more often seems apparently unsuspicious (social competence, has partner and work), and shows evidence of planning, sadism, and ritualism with the offense. The disorganized type, by contrast, shows social problems and is of below average intelligence, and the sexual homicide is impulsive and shows no or less preparation. This typology has been criticized because of its weak theoretical and empiric basis. Canter and colleagues[54] found that a (dimensional) continuum of organization could represent a more useful and empirically based application of this model.

Beauregard and Proulx[55] described 2 pathways to sexual homicide against women that show similarities with, but also differences to, the organized/disorganized typology:

- Sadistic pathway with a planned offense, more often strange victims, the use of physical restraints, and mutilation or humiliation of the victim
- Anger pathway with a nonplanned offense, no preselection of the victim, use of physical restraints, without dominant mutilation or humiliation of the victim, leaving the body at the crime scene

In a recent study, Sewall and colleagues[12] differentiated between sadistic offenders, competitively disadvantaged offenders, and so-called slashers (performing acts of mutilation, disembowelment, and depersonalization of the corpse). Most typologies have in common that they contrast a group of perpetrators with sadistic characteristics from more impulsive, reactive types. However, it should be noted from a clinical point of view that there may be many types of overlapping characteristics.

Diagnostic Dilemmas

Because sexual sadistic offenders may be reluctant to acknowledge sexual arousal attributable to sadistic fantasies or urges, which is a required motive for sexually sadistic behavior, the effectiveness of phallometric assessment has been investigated as a means of distinguishing sadistic from nonsadistic offenders. Attention has also focused on information gleaned from crime-scene behaviors of convicted offenders, which is one of the reasons why crime-scene analysis plays an important role in studies on sexual homicide.

Marshall and colleagues[24] investigated the reliability and validity of sexual sadism diagnoses in 59 male sexual offenders in Canadian prisons (41 diagnosed with sexual sadism and 18 with other DSM diagnoses [nonsadists]). Archival data indicated that sexual sadists did not differ from nonsadists on offense characteristics identified in the clinical literature as behavioral features characteristic of sexual sadism, and that nonsadistic offenders actually scored higher on some behavioral features. Moreover, sadists showed greater phallometric arousal to nonsexual violent stimuli, whereas nonsadists demonstrated greater phallometric arousal to consenting adult stimuli. The investigators concluded that nonsadists appeared more deviant than the sadists, underscoring the unreliability of a diagnosis of sexual sadism. The study findings also suggested that behavioral features thought to indicate sexual sadism may not actually distinguish between sadists and nonsadists.[24]

Although most investigators agree that sexual sadists are sexually aroused by violent or humiliating behavior (eg, Refs.[56–58]), there are conceptual differences in perspective. Some researchers have suggested that sexual arousal occurs as a result of the victim's reaction to violence or humiliating behavior,[59] and others suggest it is due to the feeling of power and control as a result of the violence inflicted (eg, Refs.[5,16]). Still others[15,60] propose that it is not the violence per se but the fear and pain produced by humiliation, degradation, and suffering that makes the sadist feel powerful and sexually aroused.

As sexual sadists are at risk for sexual offense relapses,[61,62] the need for accurate diagnoses of sexual sadism is heightened. Diagnosticians may have to rely on offenders' self-reports to confirm sadistic fantasies when there is no obvious behavioral evidence of sexual sadism. However, reliance on an individual's willingness to admit to violent sexual fantasies is problematic, given that perpetrators may be unlikely to report such fantasies.

Controversy has surrounded the proposed revisions for paraphilic diagnoses in the DSM-5.[63,64] A new diagnosis "Paraphilic Coercive Disorder," a disorder applying to men who attain sexual arousal from sexual coercion and are not sexual sadists, was proposed for inclusion in the appendix of the DSM-5.[7] Frances and Wollert[64] maintain that evaluators who tend to overclassify individuals as sexually violent predators may start to assign the diagnosis of sexual sadism to rapists more often. The investigators note that despite common factors, rape and sexual sadism differ greatly in motivation, and that only a small proportion of rapists qualify for a diagnosis of sexual sadism. First and Frances[65] noted that specific wording for differentiating rapists from sexual sadists, including the words "or behaviors" to criterion A in DSM-IV, may have resulted in forensic evaluators inappropriately concluding that a person who had committed rape would qualify for the diagnosis of a mental disorder on the basis of repeated (criminal) acts of sexual violence alone. Frances and Wollert[64] stated that the rejection by the DSM-5 Task Force of the proposal to include paraphilic coercive disorder as an official diagnosis underscores that rape is a crime and not a mental disorder.

Process of Elimination

Nonconsensual sexual acts should be differentiated from sexual arousal attributable to consensual relations that include domination. People with sexual interests in

BDSM[66] may engage in the infliction of pain, physical restraint, deliberate humiliation, and the use of fantasy or role-playing.[67,68] With consensual sadomasochism the masochist enjoys being dominated, and the infliction of pain is sexually arousing for the sadistic partner. Individuals who practice consensual sadomasochism do not victimize others, and the outcome of consensual sex acts is not typically injurious to the masochistic partner. By contrast, nonconsent of victims and personal distress are essential features in sexual sadism disorder.

Differences between DSM and ICD-10[6] criteria for sadomasochism have furthered the confusion about the term sadism. In the DSM-IV-TR, sexual sadism and sexual masochism are considered paraphilic disorders. The ICD-10 combines the conditions of sexual sadism and sexual masochism, but differentiates between sadomasochistic behaviors that are sexually motivated and those whereby violence is necessary for sexual arousal.

Comorbidities

Psychiatric disorders are prevalent in sexual offenders in forensic psychiatric settings, including Axis II disorders (paranoid personality disorder, cluster B personality disorders, and cluster C personality disorders).[69–73] In sexual homicide perpetrators, aside from paraphilia, high lifetime prevalence rates were found for substance-related disorders, sexual dysfunctions, and personality disorders such as antisocial, borderline, sadistic, and schizoid.[49]

Sexual sadism was found to be comorbid with psychopathy (eg, Ref.[74]) and shows considerable overlap with the construct of psychopathy.[75] Kirsch and Becker[76] suggested that the relationship between psychopathy and sexual sadism could be explained by emotional deficits in the ability to empathize with others, and the behavioral consequences of the condition (ie, an increased propensity for instrumental violence). More recently, Mokros and colleagues[77] reported findings in accordance with those of Kirsch and Becker[76] in a sample of 100 male forensic patients who were convicted of sexual offenses, half of whom had been diagnosed with sexual sadism. The investigators concluded that sexual sadism and psychopathy are different constructs but that are both characterized by deficit in emotional attachment. Nitschke and colleagues[78] assessed empathic capacity in 12 sexual sadists and 23 nonsadistic sexual offenders, and found no difference between the groups with respect to positive or negative stimuli. The investigators suggested that sexual sadism is not a deficit in emotional processing, but a distinct deviant pattern of sexual arousal.

Management Goals

- Reduce distress or impairment (if existent) in individuals with sexual sadism disorder.
- Reduce sexual impulsivity and/or sexual preoccupation, if sexual sadism disorder is associated with a risk for sexual offending.
- Improve control over sexual sadistic fantasies, urges, impulses, and behavior if there is a risk for sexual offending.
- Develop alternative forms of sexuality, if there is distress, impairment, and/or a risk for sexual offending.

Pharmacological Treatment Options

For medical treatment selective serotonin reuptake inhibitors, cyproterone acetate, medroxyprogesterone acetate, and gonadotropin-releasing hormone agonists have been used, depending on severity of symptoms and risk. For a detailed description the reader is referred to the article "Pharmacological Treatment of Paraphilias," by Thibaut and colleagues, elsewhere in this issue.

Nonpharmacological Treatment Options

For a detailed description of psychotherapy please see the article "Psychological Treatment of Sex Offenders: Recent Innovations," by Marshall and Marshall, elsewhere in this issue.

To the authors' knowledge there are no specific treatment programs for sexual sadistic sex offenders, and it is still controversial as to whether the psychotherapy that is applied to patients who have committed sexual offences is effective. In a forensic context, treatment intensity and interventions for patients with sexual sadism disorder depend on the risk for sexual violence, criminogenic needs (ie, sexual preoccupation), and responsivity factors (ie, psychopathy). The primary treatment goal of some cognitive-behavioral approaches, assuming unchangeable paraphilic interests, is to control sexual behavior. It has been argued that a treatment of empathy deficits could be contraindicated in sexual sadistic sex offenders because these persons would gain pleasure from the suffering of their victims and, thus, are able to take their perspective. Kingston and Yates[79] propose the use of the self-regulation model, and note that sexual sadistic offenders are often characterized by an intact self-regulation. Treatment within this model would target goals, attitudes, cognition, and behaviors that are supportive of sadistically motivated offending and less on empathy deficits or impulsivity.

Treatment Resistance, Complications, and Disease Recurrence

There is an ongoing debate regarding the possibility of changing paraphilic interests. From an empirical point of view, this issue is still open to debate. Clinically, patients report changes as well as fixed paraphilic interests across the life span. As a consequence, treatment providers should focus on individual cases to decide whether changes in paraphilic interests may be achieved. Of importance is that each decision may have strong implications: On the one hand, it might be critical to stress unchangeable paraphilic interests, because this might reduce patients' motivation for changing their sexual behavior. According to this position, treatment would rather stabilize deviant interests, and fail to address one of the most important risk factors for sexual violence. In addition, there might be a negative influence on the self-efficacy of patients and their capacity for self-control. On the other hand, the idea of changing sexual interests could overestimate the impact of treatment and lead to a waste of resources resulting from an unrealistic treatment goal.

Evaluation of Outcome, Adjustment of Treatment, and Long-term Recommendations

For the evaluation of treatment the usual dynamic risk-assessment tools (eg, the Stable 2007)[22] and therapist rating scales[80] may be used.

SUMMARY

Evaluators must differentiate sexual sadists from rapists, including looking at the viability of nonsadistic explanations for sexual violence.[64] A distinction must be made between consensual and nonconsensual sexual acts in individuals identified as sadists or masochists. Frances and Wollert[64] suggest that evaluators attempt to reduce diagnostic errors by documenting the presence of the DSM-defined required features of sexual sadism, and ruling out differential diagnoses. As noted, however, in a forensic context most sadists likely would deny being sexually excited by their victim's suffering, so other evidence may need to be relied on. Sexual sadism may be relevant in only around 10% of men who rape and in one-third of sexual homicide perpetrators. Therefore, especially in sexual homicide perpetrators, the assessment of sexual sadism is important if it has a relationship with a motivational pathway toward sexual offending.

Specific therapeutic approaches for sexual sadistic patients with a substantial risk for sexual offending focus on a reduction of sexual urges or preoccupation via lowering testosterone through medication. It will be necessary in future studies to prove the efficacy of both pharmacological and specific psychotherapeutic interventions.

REFERENCES

1. Moser C, Kleinplatz PJ. DSM-IV-TR and the paraphilias: an argument for removal. J Psychol Hum Sex 2005;17:91–109.
2. Richters J, de Visser RO, Rissel CE, et al. Demographic and psychosocial features of participants in bondage and discipline, "sadomasochism" or dominance and submission (BDSM): data from a national survey. J Sex Med 2008;5:1660–8.
3. Connolly PH. Psychological functioning of bondage/domination/sadomasochism (BDSM) practitioners. J Psychol Hum Sex 2006;18:79–120.
4. von Krafft-Ebing R. Psychopathia sexualis. Eine klinisch-forensische studie. Stuttgart (Germany): Ferdinand Enke; 1886.
5. Brittain RP. The sadistic murderer. Med Sci Law 1970;10:198–207.
6. World Health Organization. Tenth revision of the International Classification of Diseases, chapter V (F): mental and behavioural disorders. Diagnostic criteria for research. Geneva (Switzerland): World Health Organization; 1993.
7. American Psychiatric Association. Diagnostic and statistical manual of mental disorders. 5th edition. Arlington (VA): American Psychiatric Publishing; 2013. p. 685–705.
8. American Psychiatric Association. Diagnostic and statistical manual of mental disorders. 3rd edition, Revised. Washington, DC: American Psychiatric Association; 1987.
9. American Psychiatric Association. Diagnostic and statistical manual of mental disorders. 4th edition. Washington, DC: American Psychiatric Association; 1994.
10. American Psychiatric Association. Diagnostic and statistical manual of mental disorders. 4th edition, Text revision. Washington, DC: American Psychiatric Association; 2000.
11. Ressler RK, Burgess AW, Douglas JE. Sexual homicide: patterns and motives. Lexington (MA): Lexington Books; 1988.
12. Sewall LA, Krupp BA, Lalumiere M. A test of two typologies of sexual homicide. Sex Abuse 2013;25:82–100.
13. Bourget D, Bradford JM. Evidential basis for the assessment and treatment of sex offenders. Brief Treatment and Crisis Intervention 2008;8:130–46.
14. Rettenberger M, Hill A, Dekker A, et al. Genital abnormalities in early childhood in sexual homicide perpetrators. J Sex Med 2013;10:972–80.
15. Gratzer T, Bradford JM. Offender and offense characteristics of sexual sadists: a comparative study. J Forensic Sci 1995;40:450–5.
16. Dietz PE, Hazelwood RR, Warren J. The sexually sadistic criminal and his offenses. Bull Am Acad Psychiatry Law 1990;18:163–78.
17. Blumer D. Changes in sexual behavior related to temporal lobe disorders in man. J Sex Res 1970;6:173–80.

18. Siegel A. Limbic system I. Behavioral, anatomical, and physiological considerations. In: Siegel A, editor. The neurobiology of aggression and rage. Boca Raton (FL): CRC Press; 2005. p. 81–126.

19. Briken P, Habermann N, Berner W, et al. The influence of brain abnormalities on psychosocial development, criminal history and paraphilias in sexual murderers. J Forensic Sci 2005;50:1204–8.

20. Briken P, Habermann N, Berner W, et al. XYY chromosome abnormality in sexual homicide perpetrators. Am J Med Genet B Neuropsychiatr Genet 2006;141:198–200.

21. Harris A, Phenix A, Hanson RK, et al. Static-99 coding rules revised 2003. Ottawa (Canada): Department of the Solicitor General of Canada; 2003.

22. Hanson RK, Harris AJ, Scott TL, et al. Assessing the risk of sexual offenders on community supervision: the dynamic supervision project. (User report no. 2007-05). (Canada): Public Safety and Emergency Preparedness; 2007.

23. Boer DP, Hart SD, Kropp PR, et al. Manual for the Sexual Violence Risk - 20. Burnaby, B.C. Canada: Mental health, Law and Policy Institute, Simon Fraser University; 1997.

24. Marshall WL, Kennedy P, Yates P, et al. Diagnosing sexual sadism in sexual offenders: reliability across diagnosticians. Int J Offender Ther Comp Criminol 2002;46:668–77.

25. Marshall WL, Hucker SJ. Issues in the diagnosis of sexual sadism. Sexual offender treatment I. 2006. Available at: http://www.sexual-offender-treatment.org/40.html#top. Accessed January 11, 2013.

26. Nitschke J, Osterheider M, Mokros A. A cumulative scale of severe sexual sadism. Sex Abuse 2009;21:262–78.

27. Mokros A, Schilling F, Eher R, et al. The Severe Sexual Sadism Scale: cross-validation and scale properties. Psychol Assess 2012;24:764–9.

28. Nichols HR, Molinder I. Multiphasic sex inventory manual. (Available from 437 Bowes Drive, Tacoma, WA 98466). 1984.

29. Freund K. Scales for the standardized diagnostic procedure and assessment of paraphilic interests. Available at: http://individual.utoronto.ca/ray_blanchard/index_files/EPES.html. Accessed January 11, 2013.

30. Kingston DA, Seto MC, Firestone P, et al. Comparing indicators of sexual sadism as predictors of recidivism among adult male sexual offenders. J Consult Clin Psychol 2010;78:574–84.

31. Quinsey VL, Harris GT, Rice ME, et al. Violent offenders: appraising and managing risk. 2nd edition. Washington, DC: American Psychological Association; 2006.

32. Hare RD. The hare psychopathy checklist-revised. Toronto: Multi-Health Systems; 1991.

33. Hanson RK, Morton-Bourgon KE. The accuracy of recidivism risk assessments for sexual offenders: a meta-analysis of 118 prediction studies. Psychol Assess 2009;21:1–21.

34. Kingston DA, Yates PM, Firestone P, et al. Long-term predictive validity of the risk matrix 2000: a comparison with the Static-99 and the Sex Offender Risk Appraisal Guide. Sex Abuse 2008;20:466–84.

35. Koss MP, Oros CJ. Sexual Experiences Survey: a research instrument investigating sexual aggression and victimization. J Consult Clin Psychol 1982;50:455–7.

36. Koss MP, Gidycz CA, Wisniewski NR. The scope of rape: incidence and prevalence of sexual aggression and victimization in a national sample of students in higher education. J Consult Clin Psychol 1987;55:162–70.

37. Malamuth NM, Sockloskie RJ, Koss MP, et al. Characteristics of aggressors against women: testing a model using a national sample of college students. J Consult Clin Psychol 1991;59:670–81.

38. Healey J, Lussier P, Beauregard E. Sexual sadism in the context of rape and sexual homicide: An examination of crime scene indicators. Int J Offender Ther Comp Criminol 2012;57:402–24.

39. Seto MC, Lalumière ML, Harris GT, et al. The sexual responses of sexual sadists. J Abnorm Psychol 2012;121:739–53.

40. Marshall WL, Hucker SJ. Severe sexual sadism: its features and treatment. In: McAnulty RD, Burnette MM, editors. Sex and sexuality: sexual deviation and sexual offenses, vol. 3. Westport (CT): Praeger; 2006. p. 227–50.

41. Langevin R, Ben-Aron MH, Wright P, et al. The sex killer. Sex Abuse 1988;1: 263–301.

42. Hucker S, Langevin R, Dickey R, et al. Cerebral damage and dysfunction in sexually aggressive men. Sex Abuse 1988;1:33–47.

43. Harenski CL, Thornton DM, Harenski KA, et al. Increased frontotemporal activation during pain observation in sexual sadism. Arch Gen Psychiatry 2012;69: 283–92.

44. Kingston DA, Firestone P, Moulden HM, et al. The utility of the diagnosis of pedophilia. A comparison of various classification procedures. Arch Sex Behav 2007; 36:423–36.

45. Moulden HM, Firestone P, Kingston DA, et al. Recidivism in pedophiles: an investigation using different methods of defining pedophilia. J Forens Psychiatry Psychol 2009;20:680–701.

46. Krueger RB. The DSM diagnostic criteria for sexual sadism. Arch Sex Behav 2010;39:325–45.

47. Eher R, Rettenberger M, Schilling F. Psychiatrische Diagnosen von Sexualstraftätern: Eine empirische Untersuchung von 807 inhaftierten Kindesmissbrauchstätern und Vergewaltigern. [Psychiatric diagnoses of sexual offenders. An empirical study of 807 incarcerated child abuse offenders and rapists]. Z Sexualforsch 2010;23:23–35.

48. Mokros A, Schilling F, Weiss K, et al. Sadism in sexual offenders: evidence for dimensionality. Psychol Assess 2014;26:138–47.

49. Hill A, Habermann N, Berner W, et al. Sexual sadism and sadistic personality disorder in sexual homicide. J Personal Dis 2006;20:671–84.

50. Stoller R. Perversion: The Erotic Form of Hatred, Pantheon, New York, 1975.

51. Berner W, Briken P. Pleasure seeking and the aspect of longing for an object in perversion. A neuropsychoanalytical perspective. Am J Psychother 2012;66: 129–50.

52. Hill A, Habermann N, Berner W, et al. Single and multiple sexual homicide. Psychopathology 2007;40:22–8.

53. Hill A, Habermann N, Klusmann D, et al. Criminal recidivism in sexual homicide Perpetrators. Int J Offender Ther Comp Criminol 2008;52:5–20.

54. Canter DV, Alison LJ, Alison E, et al. The organized/disorganized typology of serial murder. Myth of model? Psychol Publ Pol Law 2004;10:293–320.

55. Beauregard E, Proulx J. Profiles in the offending processes of nonserial sexual murderers. Int J Offender Ther Comp Criminol 2002;46:386–99.

56. Abel GG. Paraphilias. In: Kaplan HI, Sadock BJ, editors. Comprehensive textbook of psychiatry, vol. 1, 5th edition. Baltimore (MD): Williams & Williams; 1989. p. 1069–89.

57. Knight RA, Prentky RA. Classifying sexual offenders: the development and corroboration of taxonomic models. In: Marshall WL, Law DL, Barbaree HE, editors. Handbook of sexual assault: issues, theories and treatment of the offender. New York: Plenum; 1990. p. 23–52.
58. Knight RA, Prentky RA, Cerce DD. The development, reliability, and validity of an inventory for the multidimensional assessment of sex and aggression. Crim Justice Behav 1994;21:72–94.
59. Marshall WL, Kennedy P. Sexual sadism in sexual offenders: an elusive diagnosis. Aggress Violent Behav 2003;8:1–22.
60. Richards H, Jackson RL. Behavioral discriminators of sexual sadism and paraphilia nonconsent in a sample of civilly committed sexual offenders. Int J Offender Ther Comp Criminol 2011;55(2):207–27.
61. Berner W, Berger P, Hill A. Sexual sadism. Int J Offender Ther Comp Criminol 2003;47:383–95.
62. Eher R, Schilling F, Hansmann BT. Sexual sadism and violent reoffending in sexual offenders. Paper presented at ATSA conference. October 30–November 2, 2013, Chicago, Illinois, USA.
63. Frances A. Whither DSM-V? Br J Psychiatry 2009;195:391–2.
64. Frances A, Wollert R. Sexual sadism: avoiding its misuse in sexually violent predator evaluations. J Am Acad Psychiatry Law 2012;40:409–16.
65. First MB, Frances A. Issues for DSM-V: unintended consequences of small changes: the case of paraphilias. Am J Psychiatry 2008;165:1240–1.
66. Kleinplatz P, Moser C. Toward clinical guidelines for working with BDSM clients. Contemp Sexuality 2004;38:1–4.
67. Alison L, Santtila P, Sandnabba NK, et al. Sadomasochistically oriented behavior: diversity in practice and meaning. Arch Sex Behav 2001;30:1–12.
68. Sandnabba NK, Santtila P, Alison L, et al. Demographics, sexual behaviour, family background and abuse experiences of practitioners of sadomasochistic sex: a review of recent research. Sex Relat Ther 2002;17:39–55.
69. Marshall WL. Diagnostic issues, multiple paraphilias, and comorbid disorders in sexual offenders: their incident and treatment. Aggress Behav 2007;12:16–35.
70. Dunsieth NW Jr, Nelson EB, Brusman-Lovins LA, et al. Psychiatric and legal features of 113 men convicted of sexual offences. J Clin Psychiatry 2004;65:293–300.
71. Fazel S, Sjöstedt G, Långström N, et al. Severe mental illness and risk of sexual offending in men: a case-control study based on Swedish national registers. J Clin Psychiatry 2007;68:588–96.
72. Myers WC. Juvenile sexual homicide. London: Academic Press; 2002.
73. McElroy S, Soutullo CA, Taylor P, et al. Psychiatric features of 36 men convicted of sexual offences. J Clin Psychiatry 1999;60:414–20.
74. Holt SE, Meloy JR, Strack S. Sadism and psychopathy in violent and sexually violent offenders. J Am Acad Psychiatry Law 1999;27:23–32.
75. Hare RD, Neumann CS. Psychopathy as a clinical and empirical construct. Annu Rev Clin Psychol 2008;4:217–46.
76. Kirsch LG, Becker JV. Emotional deficits in psychopathy and sexual sadism: implications of violent and sadistic behavior. Clin Psychol Rev 2007;27:904–22.
77. Mokros A, Osterheider M, Hucker SJ, et al. Psychopathy and sexual sadism. Law Hum Behav 2011;35:188–99.
78. Nitschke J, Istrefi S, Osterheider M, et al. Empathy in sexually sadistic offenders: an experimental comparison with non-sadistic sexual offenders. Int J Law Psychiatry 2012;35:165–7.

79. Kingston D, Yates P. Sexual sadism: assessment and treatment. In: Laws R, ÓDonohue WT, editors. Sexual deviance. Theory, assessment, and treatment. New York: The Guilford Press; 2008. p. 231–49.
80. Marshall WL, Marshall LE, Serran GA, et al. Rehabilitating Sexual Offenders. A Strength Based Approach. Washington, DC: American Psychological Association; 2011.

Dysfunctional Anger and Sexual Violence

A.G. Ahmed, MBBS, LLM, MSc, MPsychMed, MRCPsych, FRCPC

KEYWORDS

- Anger • Sexual violence • Sexual homicide • Treatment • Recidivism

KEY POINTS

- Anger/hostility and other negative affects are associated with sexual offending and recidivism.
- Not all sexual aggression or homicide is motivated by anger.
- Application of the existing empirical findings is limited to a specific population of sex offenders.
- Comprehensive assessment that includes anger is essential for effective treatment and risk management of some sex offenders.
- Treatment and management strategies for perpetrators of sexual violence must consider the motivations for aggression.

NATURE OF THE PROBLEM

Although there has been extensive interest in the academic research and popular discussion on the phenomenon of sexual violence and violence in general, comparatively less interest has been shown in the emotion of anger that may precede the violent behavior. Interest in examining the role of anger and other negative affects in sexual violence has increased over the past 2 decades with the introduction of the principles of relapse prevention in the treatment of sexual offenders. This model of intervention assumes an increased probability of sexual offending when the sex offender is experiencing a negative affect.[1] Subsequent empirical research has shown that negative emotional states, such as anger, anxiety, depression boredom, and frustration, may contribute to deviant sexual fantasies and offenses,[2,3] investigators and recommend that affective regulation and coping be a targeted domain in the treatment and risk management of sex offending behavior. The self-regulation model of sex offender treatment further stresses the importance of negative emotional states in the cause of deviant sexual behavior and the role of emotion, thought, and behavior modulation

No disclosures to make.

Integrated Forensic Program, Royal Ottawa Health Group, Brockville Mental Health Center (BMHC), 1804 Highway 2 East, CP/PO Box 1050, Brockville, Ontario K6V 5W7, Canada

E-mail address: ag.ahmed@theroyal.ca

Psychiatr Clin N Am 37 (2014) 231–238

http://dx.doi.org/10.1016/j.psc.2014.03.009

0193-953X/14/$ – see front matter © 2014 Elsevier Inc. All rights reserved.

in the treatment of deviant sexual behavior and sex offending and recidivism.[4,5] This article explores the key themes of anger and sexual violence, and the role of anger in classifying sex offenders and of anger and hostility in sexual recidivism.

DEFINING SEXUAL VIOLENCE AND DYSFUNCTIONAL ANGER

The World Health Organization defines sexual violence as, "any sexual act, attempt to obtain a sexual act, unwanted sexual comments or advances, or acts to traffic, or otherwise directed, against a person's sexuality using coercion, by any person regardless of their relationship to the victim, in any setting, including but not limited to home and work."[6] This definition encompasses all forms of coerced sex resulting in sexual gratification for the perpetrator, regardless of outcome for the victim, circumstances, and setting. Although sexual violence occurs worldwide, the extent of the problem is grossly underestimated because of limited research and reliance on scanty and fragmented data from police, clinical settings, and surveys. Sexual violence, like any other form of violence, is both multifactorial and multidimensional.

Anger, like anxiety and sadness, has positive and negative consequences. Although anger is an uncomfortable, aversive emotional state, sometimes people do not wish to change feeling this way,[7] and sometimes with good reason. Anger can be adaptive or functional, but it can have pernicious effects when its frequency, intensity, or duration exceeds adaptive thresholds. Excessive anger is associated with self-defeating risk-taking,[8] poor problem solving,[9] and substance use.[10] Anger leads to hostile aggression, which is the most common form of aggression, and a propensity toward aggression,[11] and is associated with marital violence, child abuse, road rage, and assault. Descriptive studies of the triggers, behaviors, targets, and outcomes of single anger episodes have identified the major characteristics of typical anger episodes and the cultural similarities among people experiencing these episodes. Violent behaviors (physical aggression) were reported in 10% of episodes, and approximately half of the individuals experiencing these episodes reported that the effects of the anger on their relationships were positive.[12,13] From a cultural perspective, Kassinove and colleagues[13] compared American and Russian samples and found no significant differences in the components of the anger episode. Although anger is often a motivated action, excessive or inappropriate anger may be a symptoms of several of the existing disorders in the *Diagnostic and Statistical Manual of Mental Disorders* (Fifth Edition). Even though it is associated with deviant sexual, the emotion is not listed among the diagnostic criteria for any of the paraphilias in the diagnostic manual.[14]

DYSFUNCTIONAL ANGER IN SEXUAL FANTASIES AND OFFENDING BEHAVIORS

In a study of the relationship between conflict, affective states, and particular sexual behaviors (fantasies and masturbatory activities during these fantasies), McKibben and colleagues[15] had 13 rapists and 9 pedophiles in a treatment program complete a "fantasy report" every 2 days for 60 days. The fantasy report is a self-assessment method specifically the investigators developed to assess the frequency of deviant and nondeviant fantasies, sexual behaviors, presence of interpersonal conflict, and affective components.

Fantasy Report Self-Assessments

The rapists reported experiencing more negative moods and the presence of conflicts associated with overwhelming deviant sexual fantasies and increased masturbatory activities during these fantasies. Furthermore, the emotions most frequently reported by rapists after conflicts were loneliness, humiliation, anger, and feelings of inadequacy and rejection. The investigators did not find an association between affective components and nondeviant sexual behaviors in the rapists, suggesting that negative affect may not be associated with all deviant sexual fantasies.

The pedophile subgroup also only showed a significant relationship between negative affect and deviant sexual fantasies. These data suggest that, in sexual offenders, negative affect is a crucial component in the chain that leads to deviant sexual behaviors. In a comparative study of the temporal relationship between negative affect and deviant sexual behavior among convicted pedophiles and rapists and men convicted of nonsexual violence, pedophiles reported that feelings of anger, depressed mood, and rejection by a woman, and arguments with a spouse were more likely related to pedophilic fantasies than fantasies about adults.[16] Although Looman[17] hypothesizes, based on these findings, that deviant sexual fantasies help the offenders cope with negative affect, others argue that because of inherent limitations of studies beyond the scope of these articles, these findings only suggest an association between negative moods and reported fantasies.[18]

Sexual Fantasy Function Model

Finally, using qualitative research methodology and multiple sources of data on sex offenders from 3 treatment sites (a community sex offender treatment program, forensic outpatient clinic, and prison sex offender treatment program), Gee and colleagues[19] developed the Sexual Fantasy Function Model. This model identified the 4 functions of sexual fantasies as affective regulation, sexual arousal regulation, coping, and modeling experience. These qualitative studies of the negative affect (eg, anger, anxiety, and depression) associated with deviant and nondeviant sexual fantasies and sexual behavior during deviant sexual fantasies, reported by convicted sex offenders in different treatment settings, are only of limited value in understanding how to treat negative affect in sexual offenders.

Empirical Research on Sexual Offending

The relationship between negative and actual sexual offending has been the subject of empirical research, and the findings have been fairly consistent. Studies of stages of progression in pathways to sex offending among incarcerated sex offenders with child victims have revealed that negative affect was associated with either the beginning (proximal) of the sequence of the behavioral, cognitive, or emotive process, resulting in the actual offending act, or at the end during act itself (distal).[20,21] In a study of recidivism among over 400 sex offenders (208 recidivists vs 201 nonrecidivists) that used multiple sources of data (self-report measures, file information, and collateral information from community supervisors), recidivists showed increases in subjective negative affect proximal to reoffending.[22] Anger and problems with anger expression have been found to be common in high-risk reoffending situations by male sex offenders undergoing outpatient individual or group therapy.[23]

Hostility, an attitude of resentment, suspiciousness, and bitterness,[24] and the desire to get revenge or have a destructive outlet for one's anger[25] have been the focus of empirical exploration to determine the cause of sexual offending. Hall and Hirschman[26] suggested that hostility, a form of negative affect, herald and facilitate sexual aggression, whereas empathy and guilt impede feelings of hostility. The sex offenders' feelings of hostility and the associated deficient sexual and aggressive inhibitory control are attributed to poor socialization.[27] Although earlier studies[28,29] did not reveal a significant association between hostility and the degree of violence in the offenders' last offense, the number of prior violent/nonviolent convictions, or the degree of aggression in psychiatric patients, more recent studies have consistently shown that higher levels of victim-specific and general hostility were associated with sex offending.[30–32]

Sexual Reoffending

These studies have also shown a consistent association between anger and hostility and sexual reoffending.[30–32] In a 2005 study of 656 convicted male sex offenders attending a sexual behavior clinic, Firestone and colleagues[30] found a significant association between hostility and having prior violent charges, use of violence in the index sexual offense, sexual recidivism, and violent recidivism. These investigators reported that hostility was also "significantly associated with recidivism in intrafamilial and extrafamilial child molesters, but not in rapists or mixed offenders."[30]

DYSFUNCTIONAL ANGER IN SEXUAL HOMICIDE

The findings of empirical study of the pathways to sexual homicide using diverse methods in different samples of sex offenders have consistently shown anger to be an important motivation. Anger as a galvanizing and action-oriented emotion associated with aggressive sexual behavior may result in serious bodily injury to and even death of the victim. Homicides occurring while the offender is experiencing pre–crime state intense anger are commonly described as occurring through the "anger pathway," and are still classified as sexual homicides even if the primary motivation is anger/rage rather than sexual arousal. This distinction becomes important in separating the "anger motivation pathway" from other pathways (sadistic motivation pathway and sexual motivation pathway), to sexual homicide.[33–35]

Different types of dysfunctional anger exist, and awareness of the type patients are presenting with in a clinical setting is germane to the assessment and treatment of the primary diagnosis and the management of the associated risk.[36] Grubin[37] noted that many of the sexual murderers in his study overcontrolled their anger. These individuals may experience high anger arousal and are aware of it. They do not usually, however, express their anger outwardly, either with assertiveness or aggression. They may occasionally lose control and express their anger outwardly by yelling, throwing, or damaging property. When they do lose control, they immediately apologize and fear reprisal. These clients may experience alternating episodes of depression and overcontrolled anger. The anger episodes are ruminative and usually last a day or longer. Individuals in this group are similar to those high in anger-control in Spielberger's[38] model and those of the Suppressed Dysfunctional Anger type.[36] The high anger inhibition may be as problematic as the poorly controlled anger seen in the impulsively aggressive individual.[36,39]

The sudden release of overcontrolled anger and aggression is a possible explanation for the excessive use of force by perpetrators and the disproportionately excessive injuries experienced by the victims in certain cases of sexual homicide.[40] Blackburn[41] classified the overcontrolled offender into 2 types: the "conforming type," characterized by sociability, conformity, and denial of anger, and the "inhibited type," characterized by the verbalization of strong subjective anger experience, a rumination tendency, and intense levels of anger but poor expression.[42]

Catathymia, a psychodynamic concept proposed by Wertham in 1937,[40,43] has been advanced as a possible explanation for some sexual homicides.[44–46] Catathymia is characterized by episodic severe and out-of-character violence associated with quasi-delusional rigid thinking that occurs after extreme emotional tension, and is followed by calm and superficial normalcy.

In exploring the functional role of anger in sexual violence, Zillmann[47] argues that sex and aggression are severally interdependent, and anger arousal and sexual arousal are physiologically linked through endocrine system, autonomic nervous system, and the central nervous system (via the limbic system structures, amygdala, and the septal area). In keeping with the excitation-transfer theory, the residual excitation of one arousal state (anger) can continue and strengthen another arousal state (sexual). Money[48] hypothesized that because of the proximity in the limbic system structures of the brain and the knitting of neural connections, the sexual arousal system and the process responsible for aggression may be activated at the same.

Sexual homicides occurring through the sadistic motivation pathway are not primarily motivated by anger, but rather by sexual excitement caused by the psychological or physical suffering (including humiliation) of the victim, which some researchers argue is primarily related to "the quest for control and domination of the victim."[49–51] Inflicting suffering on the victim (not death) is the primary motivation, with domination and control as the primary or secondary goals, and the aggression is instrumental rather than anger-motivated. Similarly for sexual murders occurring through the sexual motivation pathway, the primary motivation is sex and the aggression is instrumental rather than anger-motivated or anger-reactive.[52]

SUMMARY AND IMPLICATIONS FOR CLINICAL PRACTICE AND FUTURE RESEARCH

This article examines how anger and hostility are related to sexual offending. The role of anger in deviant sexual fantasies and offending, sexual recidivism, and sexual homicide are specifically reviewed. Although the findings in the sex offender literature have several limitations (eg, small sample sizes, male gender only, type II error, non-randomization, retrospective nature) and are not conclusive, they suggest a strong association between anger/hostility and sex offending, anger-motivated sexual homicide, and recidivism. These observations are beneficial in the assessment and treatment of convicted and incarcerated sex offenders, which is the focus of most of the empirical work reviewed in this article. The application of these findings to qualitatively different populations (eg, female sex offenders or sex offenders not yet arrested) is questionable and must occur with caution. The findings support that a treatment and risk management approach should include the assessment and treatment of dysfunctional anger. Finally, future research will benefit from a more precise definition of the concept, the use of a non–sex offender control group, prospective design, and a more systematic examination of the role of anger in sexual offending.

REFERENCES

1. Pithers WD, Kashima KM, Cumming GF, et al. Relapse prevention of sexual aggression. In: Prentky RA, Quinsey QL, editors. Human sexual aggression: current perspectives, vol. 528. New York: New York Academy of Sciences; 1988. p. 244–60.
2. Serran G, Marshall L. Coping and mood in sexual offending. In: Marshall W, Fernandez Y, Marshall LE, et al, editors. Sexual offending treatment: controversial issues. West Sussex (England): John Wiley & Sons. Ltd; 2006. p. 109–24.
3. Ward T, Hudson S. A self-regulation model of relapse prevention. In: Laws DR, Hudson SM, Ward T, editors. Remaking relapse prevention with sex offenders: a sourcebook. Thousand Oaks (CA): Sage Publications; 2000. p. 79–101.
4. Cortoni F, Marshall W. Sex as a coping strategy and its relationship to juvenile and intimacy offenders. Sex Abuse 2001;38:61–79.
5. Ward T, Hudson SM, Marshall WL. The abstinence violation effect in child molesters. Behaviour Research and Therapy 1994;32(4):431–7.

6. Krug E, Mercy J, Dahlberg L, et al, editors. World report on violence and health. Geneva (Switzerland): World Health Organization; 2002.
7. Scherer KR, Wallbott HG. Evidence for the universality and cultural variation of differential emotional response patterns. J Pers Soc Psychol 1994;67(1): 55–65.
8. Leith KP, Baumeister RF. Why do bad moods increase self-defeating behavior? Emotion, risk taking, and self-regulation. Journal of Personality and Social Psychology 1996;71:1250–67.
9. Novaco RW. The function and regulation of the arousal of anger. Am J Psychiatry 1976;133:1124–8.
10. Deffenbacher JL. Cognitive-relaxation and social skills treatments of anger: a year later. J Couns Psychol 1988;35:234–6.
11. Baumeister R, Smart L, Boden J. Relation of threatened egotism to violence and aggression: the dark side of high self-esteem. Psychol Rev 1996;103:5–33.
12. Averill JR. Studies on anger and aggression. Implications for theories of emotion. Am Psychol 1983;38:1145–60.
13. Kassinove H, Sukhodolsky DG, Tystsarev DV, et al. Self-reported constructions of anger episodes in Russia and America. J Soc Behav Pers 1997;12:301–24.
14. American Psychiatric Association. Diagnostic and statistical manual of mental disorders. 5th edition. Arlington (VA): American Psychiatric Association; 2013.
15. McKibben A, Proulx J, Lusignan R. Relationships between conflict, affect and deviant sexual behaviors in rapists and pedophiles. Behav Res Ther 1994; 32(5):571–5.
16. Looman J. Sexual fantasies of child molesters. Can J Behav Sci 1995;27: 321–32.
17. Looman J. Mood, conflict, and deviant sexual fantasies. In: Schwartz BK, editor. The sex offender: theoretical advances, treating populations and legal development. Vol. 3.1999.
18. McCoy K, Fremouw W. The relation between negative affect and sexual offending: A critical review. Clinical Psychology Review 2010;30:317–25.
19. Gee D, Ward T, Eccleston L. The function of sexual fantasies for sexual offenders: A preliminary model. Behaviour Change 2003;20:44–60.
20. Hudson S, Ward T, McCormack J. Offense pathways in sexual offenders. Journal of Interpersonal Violence 1999;14:779–97.
21. Ward T, Hudson S, Marshall W. Cognitive distortions and affective deficits in sex offenders: a cognitive deconstructionist interpretation. Sex Abuse 1995;7:67–83.
22. Hanson RK, Harris A. Where should we intervene? Dynamic predictors of sexual offense recidivism. Criminal Justice and Behaviour 2000;27:6–35.
23. Price D. Relapse prevention and risk reduction: results of client identification of high risk situations. Sex Addict Compulsivity 1999;6:221–52.
24. Buss A, Perry M. The aggression questionnaire. Personality and Social Psychology 1992;63:452–9.
25. Mikulincer M. Adult attachment style and individual differences in functional versus dysfunctional experiences of anger. Journal of Personality and Social Psychology 1998;74:513–24.
26. Hall GC, Hirschman R. Toward a theory of sexual aggression: a quadripartite model. J Consult Clin Psychol 1991;59:643–69.
27. Marshall WL, Barbaree HE. An integrated theory of the etiology of sexual offending. In: Marshall WL, Laws DR, Barbaree HE, editors. Handbook of sexual assault: Issues, theories, and treatment of the offender. New York: Plenum; 1990. p. 257–75.

28. Edmunds G. The predictive validity of the Buss-Durkee Inventory. Journal of Clinical Psychology 1976;32:818–20.
29. Holland TR, Levi M, Beckett GE. Ethnicity, criminality, and the Buss-Durkee Hostility Inventory. Journal of Personality Assessment 1983;47:375–9.
30. Firestone P, Nunes KL, Moulden BA, et al. Hostility and recidivism in sexual offenders. Arch Sex Behav 2005;34(3):277–83.
31. Lee JK, Pattison P, Jackson HJ, et al. The general, common, and specific factors of psychopathology for different types of paraphilias. Crim Justice Behav 2001; 28:227–66.
32. Marshall WL, Moulden H. Hostility toward women and victim empathy in rapists. Sex Abuse 2001;13:249–55.
33. Cusson M, Proulx J. The motivation and crime career of sexual murderers. In: Proulx J, Beauregard E, Cusson M, et al, editors. Sexual murders: a comparative analysis and new perspectives. Chichester (United Kingdom): Wiley; 2007. p. 142–55.
34. Kerr KJ, Beech AR, Murphy D. Sexual homicide: definition, motivation and comparison with other forms of sexual offending. Aggress Violent Behav 2013;18(1): 1–10.
35. Proulx J. Sexual murderers: theories, assessment and treatment. Correctional Service Canada Web site. Available at: http://www.csc-scc.gc.ca/research/shp2007-paraphil12-eng.shtml#archived. Accessed March 2, 2014.
36. Ahmed AG, Kingston DA, DiGiuseppe R, et al. Developing a clinical typology of dysfunctional anger. J Affect Disord 2013;136(1):139–48.
37. Grubin D. Sexual murder. British Journal of Psychiatry 1994;165:624–9.
38. Spielberger CD. Manual for the State-Trait Anger Expression Inventory–2. Odessa (FL): Psychological Assessment Resources; 1999.
39. Davey L, Day A, Howells K. Anger, over-control and serious violent offending. Aggress Violent Behav 2005;10(5):624–35.
40. Kerr KJ, Beech AR, Murphy D. Sexual homicide: Definition, motivation and comparison with other forms of sexual offending. Aggression and Violent Behavior 2013;18:1–10.
41. Blackburn R. The psychology of criminal conduct: Theory, research and practice. Toronto: Wiley; 1993.
42. Tice DM, Baumeister RF. Controlling anger: Self-induced emotion change. In: Wegner DM, Pennebaker JW, editors. Handbook of mental control. Englewood Cliffs, NJ: Prentice Hall; 1993. p. 393–409.
43. Wertham F. The catathymic crisis: A clinical entity. Archives of Neurology and Psychiatry 1937;37:974–8.
44. Revitch E, Schlesinger L. The psychopathology of homicide. Springfield, IL: Charles C Thomas; 1981.
45. Schlesinger LB. Sexual homicide: Differentiating catathymic and compulsive murders. Aggression and Violent Behavior 2007;12:242–56.
46. Meloy JR. The nature and dynamics of sexual homicide: An integrative review. Aggression and Violent Behavior 2000;5:1–22.
47. Zillmann D. Aggression and sex: independent and joint operations. In: Wagner H, Manstead A, editors. Handbook of social psychophysiology. Chichester (United Kingdom): Wiley; 1989. p. 229–60.
48. Money J. Forensic sexology: paraphilic serial rape (biastophilia) and lust murder (erotophonophilia). Am J Psychother 1990;44:26–36.
49. Ressler RK, Burgess AW, Douglas JE. Sexual homicide: patterns and motives. New York: Lexington; 1988.

50. Revitch E, Schlesinger L. Sex murder and sex aggression: phenomenology, psychopathology and prognosis. Springfield (IL): Charles C Thomas; 1989.
51. Spielberger CD. Manual for the state trait anger expression inventory. Odessa (FL): Psychological Assessment Resources; 1988.
52. Beech A, Oliver C, Fisher D, et al. STEP 4: The sex offender treatment programme in prison: Addressing the offending behaviour of rapists and sexual murderers. London, England: Her Majesty's Prison Service; 2005.

Ethics and the Treatment of Sexual Offenders

Mansfield Mela, MBBS, MSc[a],
A.G. Ahmed, MBBS, LLM, MSc, MPsychMed, MRCPsych, FRCPC[b],*

KEYWORDS

- Sex offenders • Ethics • Treatment • Consent • Confidentiality circle • Dual agency

KEY POINTS

- Standardization of assessment procedures is essential.
- Second opinions may be necessary in treating resistance cases and consenting procedures.
- Current evidence of effectiveness is imperative in pharmacologic and psychosocial treatment.
- Limits of acceptable behavior in the patient–therapist relationship depend on the balance of best interests of the patient and public safety.
- Professionals should be aware of the implications of court-ordered mandated treatment.
- Sex offender reporting and notification laws have produced mixed outcomes on treatment access and public safety.

INTRODUCTION

Current clinical practices implicated as a source of ethical dilemmas in sex offender treatment are those that concern the superiority of public safety over the interests of patient, clients, or offenders (hereon referred as to *patients*). When pitched against the best interests of patients, the interest of patient stands no chance if it is considered an either or matter.[1] Restricting the goals of treatment to the sole purpose of reducing the risk of recidivism not only limits the value of but also potentially replaces the traditional ethically informed therapeutic relationship and the joint collaborative goals that flow from it. Usually in a relationship, such as exists between therapist and patient, the voice of the patient is encouraged and is necessary in setting treatment goals and monitoring progress. When coercion is perceived or experienced, treatment is estimated as superficial, short lived, and lacking commitment. In

[a] Department of Psychiatry, Faculty of Medicine, University of Saskatchewan, Saskatoon, Saskatchewan, Canada; [b] Divisions of Forensic Psychiatry and Addiction and Mental Health, Department of Psychiatry, University of Ottawa and the Royal Ottawa Health Care Group, Ottawa, Ontario, Canada
* Corresponding author.
E-mail address: ag.ahmed@theroyal.ca

Psychiatr Clin N Am 37 (2014) 239–250
http://dx.doi.org/10.1016/j.psc.2014.03.008
0193-953X/14/$ – see front matter © 2014 Elsevier Inc. All rights reserved.

involuntary settings, as exist in civil commitment of sex offenders, a therapist's values and goals of public safety assume a more important influence. Some of the ethical moral and legal implications arising from civil commitment include "co-optation of medical authority to legitimate commitment based upon non-medical classifications, ex post facto application of civil commitment statutes to offenders who committed crimes decades earlier, admissibility of treatment records during a civil commitment hearing, and the likelihood of lifetime commitment that results from a finding of future dangerousness."[2] This conflict arises by virtue of treatment goals and values that are predetermined and enforced on a patient rather than self-generated collaboratively in therapy with the patient. Intrinsically derived motivations yield positive behavioral changes, such as better learning, performance, and well-being, as well as longer-lasting results than motivations derived externally.[3] If ethical guidelines recognize the vulnerabilities of sex offenders, therapists' conduct should consider the imbalances of power. Responding adequately without coercion and rapidly with no prejudice is an essential ingredient for navigating the therapeutic relationship and its perceived or real ethical conflict.

Understanding the ethical issues in sex offender treatment requires a summary of the distinct nature of the interventions. First, a diagnosable mental disorder leads to criminal offending affecting a wide range of victims, including children. Adopting a caring approach and providing sex offenders with or without a diagnosable mental disorder (paraphilia) treatment and rehabilitation have been debated extensively.[4,5] Sentiments fly high creating an avenue for conflict in ethics. The extent and contrast of the treatment approaches, content, and delivery compared with the best interest principles and autonomy create an ethical dilemma.[6] Should sex offenders be considered ill and in need of treatment or subject to only punishment for their offenses? Should voluntariness determine the mode of treatment or is there a place for compulsory treatment? Are resistance to disclosure, delay in accepting responsibility, and rationalization for offenses evidence of poor treatment engagement and thus support for punishment approaches? Does castration count as treatment if it offers the best control of offending? These questions require the balancing act that ethical practice demands. The values that delineate boundaries of permissible behavior in a patient–therapist relationship are shaped by the conceptualization of the nature of the problem experienced by the sex offender.[7]

CONCEPTUALIZATION OF SEX OFFENDERS AND TREATMENT

Whether sex offending is a disorder or a choice has received varying reviews.[8] Even paraphilia, previously referred to as sexual deviance, was unclassified as a disorder. Termed perversions, they have been described as inherently fuzzy and controversial.[9] The nosologic place of paraphilias is uncertain.[9,10] What is known is the relevance of sexual deviance as a significant risk factor in sexual offending and recidivism, thus the need for treatment.[11] That knowledge and the acceptance of aspects of sexual offending arising from a disorder influence the concepts and delivery of treatment. Sexual behavior disorder, sexual deviance, and paraphilia are used to identify the disorder component of sexual offending. Currently, treatment has been directed at eliciting treatable parts of the disorder to limit offending.[12] The primary goal of traditional mental health treatment is generally to reduce suffering by the patient and almost always promotes the best interests of the patient. In certain situations these goals may be at loggerheads with the wider goals of public protection. Most, if not all, sex offender treatment providers do not hesitate to completely excise guidance or strategies for a sex offender to avoid detection from the armamentarium of treatment.

This is true even when a sex offender determines that such knowledge is a best interest goal of some sort. This extreme example demonstrates the stake of balancing best interest and public safety in treatment, but less egregious examples are the bedrock of ethical dilemmas. To successfully negotiate this sensitive bind is to consider the nonexclusive nature of treatment goals and to adopt essential safeguards as the guiding principles in treatment programs. The ethical guidelines for dealing with dual agency are far from settled and there may be professional and regional differences in the codes of practice. To ensure approaches that are consistent, transferable, and ethically universal, the Association for the Treatment of Sexual Abusers published a professional code of ethics and revised it in 2001. The guidelines go so far as including a mechanism by which ethical breaches can be reported, investigated, and sanctioned (**Table 1**).[5]

Furthermore, any informed discussion of the ethical issues in the treatment of sex offenders must distinguish between the 2 concepts of *treatment as punishment* and *treatment of the punished*.[13] Although treatment of offenders serving punishment adheres strictly to the ethical principles of beneficence (nonmaleficence), treatment as punishment (eg, court-ordered sex offender program) often violates these principles. **Table 2** compares these concepts with punishment.

Table 1
Stages of treatment and ethical issues that arise in the stages

Stages of Treatment	Relevant Ethical Themes
Conceptualization	• Choice vs disorder • Punishment vs treatment • Public safety vs individual rights • In custody vs out of custody
Assessment	• Dual agency • Phallometric testing • Disclosure of other offenses and reporting requirement • Denial of responsibility for the offense • Concealment
General treatment	• Interdisciplinary treatment team differing principles • Multiprofessional treatment team differing approaches • Length of sentence/treatment • Motivation for treatment • Hybrid orders • Responsivity • Training • Expertise/integrity • Gender and boundary violations
Pharmacologic treatment	• Choice of pharmaceutical agent • Receptor base • Chemical castration • Supervision and medication treatment
Psychosocial treatment	• Autobiography and offender victimization • Crime cycle and relapse prevention • High-risk situations • Integrity of treatment program
Others	• Sex offender registry • Employment and exposure to vulnerable persons • Consent to be research subject • Risk, need, and responsivity principles

Table 2
Characteristics of treatment of the punished, treatment as punishment, and punishment concepts

Characteristics and Values	Treatment of the Punished (eg, Treatment of a Medical Condition)	Treatment as Punishment (eg, Court-Ordered Sex Offender Program)	Punishment
Purpose of intervention	Well-being of offender	Public safety (retribution and incapacitation are of equal or more significance than rehabilitation)	Only rehabilitation is in offender's interest Deterrence, restitution, and incapacitation are in the interest of public safety
Patient's autonomy	Respects the offender's independence	Curtailment of the offender's liberty	Deprives the offender of liberty, life, or property
Confidentiality	Respects the offender's privacy	Limited confidentiality as requirement of treatment	Public safety
Beneficence	Focus on sole offender's well-being	Focus on public safety and violation	Public safety
Nonmaleficence	Adhere with only few necessary exceptions	Breaches are routine and regarded as necessary and desirable	Breaches are routine and regarded as necessary and desirable
Veracity	Treatment as treatment	Punishment disguised as treatment	Punishment as punishment

A careful analysis reveals that sex offender programs by their design have characteristics and values that are implicitly or explicitly similar to those of punishment than traditional treatment in mental health. This is necessarily so because the primary interest in these programs is the community, not the sex offender. Mental health clinicians providing this treatment and the associated infringements of the traditional ethical values are sanctioned by legal bodies (courts, parole boards, and so forth) and the community at large. That is, the planned infringement of these ethical principles and values are good for the society. The acknowledgment by the clinicians and disclosure to the offender and the community that treatment is used justifiably as punishment help set the stage for more pragmatic ethics that are specific to sex offender program and respect for sex offenders' rights.

BIOPSYCHOSOCIAL ASSESSMENT

Investigations of paraphilia in sex offenders present a string of ethical issues. The clinician assessor serves a dual role of identifying clinical features that may be targets for treatment, including assessment of substance use and its relationship to offending, impulsivity, and power and control difficulties. Components of the assessment are relevant for planning treatment but the inclusion in the assessment battery of functional analysis, performance-based measures, use of measures for treatment readiness, and the use of self-report questionnaires incur ethical queries.[14] Sexual deviance and compulsivity are treatable dynamic risk factors but assessing their presence in a particular sex offender may also uncover sexual behaviors and crimes hitherto not reported. The offender may present a concealed aspect of the past history and the assessor could be left disbelieving the account. Alternatively, revelation of unreported and unprosecuted offenses requires that certain types of offenses that expose victims, especially young victims, to future risk may need to be reported. Undoubtedly such dilemmas have led to ethical difficulties.[4,5] In a version of this dilemma when even adults may be at risk, ethical issues arose in a case when a dangerous sex offender revealed in an assessment the intention to pick up, rape, torture, and kill certain victims. The resulting saga was concluded in the legal arena with some guidelines under which reporting may be allowed ethically.[15] The other role served during assessment concerns detection of risk prevention factors in which legal remedies predominate to the detriment of clinical measures.[6,16]

Assessment is made more challenging by concerns about the method of measuring deviant arousal to sexual stimuli. Images or sound bites used to estimate the level and type of deviation have fallen out of favor with authorities. They are considered pornographic; so, in the case of a phallometric (plethysmography) laboratory in possession of nude pictures of underage persons, threats of prosecution either led to changes in the procedure or altogether canceling the procedure. Children or their parents are not legally considered consenting to the use of those pictures.[17] The use of polygraph by some laboratories leaves questions of additional reported victims, ability to pass the test, and both the control question test and the guilty knowledge test divide, which remain unanswered. Reliability and discriminant and predictive validity of phallometric assessments are not standardized across laboratories. The stimuli are varied and there was a great deal of heterogeneity in methodologies across 48 laboratories in North America reported.[18] If the newer nonvisually explicit methods do not adequately identify deviation, poor characterization of offenders ensues; thus, remaining untreatable is a possibility. It has been proposed that in certain offenders, desensitization to pornographic material diminishes the ability of the regular images in picking up deviancy.[17] To combat a high threshold for arousal, a virtual laboratory has been proposed. Virtual images of human caricatures or dolls are proposed as more effective stimuli. Virtual immersion with virtual naked models is the method by which paraphilic sexual preferences are identified and measured.[19] With laws against child pornography, it is unlikely that the new approach will be directed at those pedophiles who require a high intensive stimuli. The impasse in assessment and accurate characterization of the disorders are unresolved. Unfortunately, sometimes and for appropriate management, self-disclosure cannot be relied on.

Sex offenders who require blood tests for different investigations may opt out of completing the procedure. Exerting their rights to autonomy may compromise relevant components of the assessments. Knowledge of alcohol and drug use, endocrinological disorders contributing to sexual offending, and ensuring safety of any treatment depend on such tests. Proceeding without basic or specialized blood test may be considered ethical as long as it is balanced by a second opinion from another colleague, determined from a capacitous decision, and contemporaneously documented.

TREATMENT MODELS AND TEAMS

The treatment offered to sex offenders has been attacked as a form of brain washing, outside the realm of psychological interventions.[4] This is said to occur more so when it is deduced that an offender is not motivated. Steps to engage the offender and strategies to enhance compliance fall short of voluntary treatment by the standards of some critics. Specialized skills and training are the essential remedies to this quandary. When the dignity and autonomy of sex offenders are upheld and respected, it is easier to see how the use of motivational inducements is not incompatible with treatment principles. Under the clout of respect for the offender, resistance can be safely reduced and acknowledgment of the different defense mechanisms paves the way to guiding the offender. Through these initiatives and applying the values of respect and individuality, offenders can accept responsibility for their offense.

Treatability is debated in the area of sex offender effectiveness in care. Recovery is an up-and-coming yet common theme in other areas of forensic mental health but its use is not yet prominent in the sex offender treatment area. It may be bedeviled by misconceptions and misinformation on the pattern, nature, course, and recidivism of sex offending behavior. Examples of ethical concerns include resolving confidentiality in treatment. Consider a set of twin sex offenders in treatment. By nature of the gene environment, interactions leading to the criminal activity or paraphilia (if the activities have not led to a legal breach or charges) are expected to be prominent. Confidentiality and privacy in their strictest sense are not maintained or safeguarded from one twin to the other. A similar dilemma can occur when family members have the same need for treatment at the same time or sometime after one another. Safeguarding confidentiality can be achieved by conceptualizing the circle of confidentiality, how wide it is, those in it, and those who are on a need-to-know basis.[20]

The process and content of treatment as well as differences between the approaches used for male and female offenders have raised ethical concerns. Not only do female and male sex offenders differ on numerous psychological, life-stressor, and sexual variables but also approaches are different.[21] Models of treatment prescribe multiple professionals involved in delivering treatment to sex offenders. Questions about sharing of information and maintaining confidentiality not only make treatment safe but also are affected by the different ethical codes and standards of the several professionals on the team.[5] The specialization and training requirement for those who treat sex offenders vary from site to site. Improved outcomes are associated with specialization of programs.[22] The same has not been proved for the specialization of therapists, even though general basic training requirements are proposed. Specialized training and maintenance of certification are strongly recommended for those working with sex offenders. Enforcing such standards has not been possible, and that is ethically unsettling, especially when recommendations from these professionals form the significant consideration for decisions on reintegration. Preferred location of treatment, hospital, correctional, and outpatient settings all have advantages and disadvantages that seem to be missing parts of the treatment puzzle.

Certification of professionals' continued professional education to maintain such certification is an essential part of resolving the ethical quandary. Precertification through selection is an area of evolution. Guidelines exist to assist in the selection of clinicians and therapists with the right experience. Selection of more inquisitive professionals rather than those whose beliefs and behaviors focus only on the agenda to stop all offending can make a difference in treatment and supervision.[23] Adhering to models of treatment with evidence of their success in rehabilitation should be promoted to minimize the differing characteristics and intentions of professionals in treatment programs. Standardization of treatment ensures comparable efforts and guarantees similar results but responding to the deficits unique to individuals should guide the level of flexibility needed in each program. Treatment should be available locally so that the capacity to conduct treatment can be considered in the context of human resource planning. Also, planning reintegration where services for follow-up exist is ethically competent and likely to ensure continuity, a necessary aspect of ethical treatment of multiple demands and multifactorial disorders common among sex offenders.

Conflicting expectations, standards of care, and value systems form the basis for ethical dilemmas. In sex offender treatment, discomfort may arise in accepting acts of violation as disorders; a choice of one disposal means from another in those who have completed treatment may be unclear. Disagreement even among professionals on diagnosis, treatment effectiveness, and recidivism are common. Concern arises as to how fairness can be maintained when advancing the rights of an offender in recognition of the safety of the public.

Dimensions of delivery and model of care, including caseload estimates, present varying ethical issues. Episodic treatment occurs in institutions. Maintaining gains made may be interrupted when successfully treated offenders transition to the community, a new environment with a new set of professionals. Long-term longitudinal approaches for accountability and supervision may be lost. Current measures, correctional supervision during parole, and probation as well as registration with a sex offender registry fall short in maintaining treatment gains.

Multidisciplinary and interdisciplinary treatment models present challenges when professionals from different disciplines desire to adhere to different guidelines according to their baseline ethics and codes. The overlap in and differences between these principles can easily translate into ethical breaches. Careful consideration is needed to ensure a smooth interprofessional relationship to minimize confusion in offenders seeking treatment. Many professionals may feel the need to obtain different informed consent from offenders. Stigmatization enhanced by such procedures is not unimaginable.

INFORMED CONSENT

At its core, the discussion that leads to an informed consent should include "the patient's diagnosis, if known; the nature and purpose of a proposed treatment or procedure; the risks and benefits of a proposed treatment or procedure; alternatives (regardless of their cost or the extent to which the treatment options are covered by health insurance); the risks and benefits of the alternative treatment or procedure; and the risks and benefits of not receiving or undergoing a treatment or procedure. In turn, your patient should have an opportunity to ask questions to elicit a better understanding of the treatment or procedure, so that he or she can make an informed decision to proceed or to refuse a particular course of medical intervention."[24] The choices of treatment are sometimes negated in high-risk situations. A sex offender determined to require injectable antiandrogens may object to the libido reduction associated with lack of pleasure. Ethical considerations may bow to the legal premise of safety, and offenders have found themselves in a bind, including deciding whether to be released as asexual or to be sexual and incarcerated. This is a prominent ethical issue for the clinician and society as well.

BIOLOGIC/PHARMACOLOGIC TREATMENT

Since it has been shown that castration produced acceptable recidivism rates among sex offenders, controversy in the use of pharmacologic agents has muddied the biologic treatment arena.[25] Some US states have passed legislation authorizing chemical as well as physical castration. Directed at public safety, the ethical issues brought by these practices include giving offenders no options and violation of the constitutional rights of offenders.[26] Over the past 2 or 3 decades, advancements in knowledge of mechanisms of mental disorder as well as clinical trials of medications have tempered the plight of medications and sex offending. Choice of medication over self-control has been debated based on the conceptualization of the problem. An algorithm by the World Federation of Societies of Biological Psychiatry for the biologic treatment of sex offenders has helped in standardizing treatment.[27,28] A stage-wise approach based on risk levels and close monitoring of side effects make treatment with pharmacologic agents refined and easily rationalized. Concerns exist as to how compliance can be ensured and whether persons released on medications are voluntarily taking them or being forced to accept them. Without an option for incarceration, a few sex offenders may accept medications.[26] Ethical issues on voluntariness, a crucial aspect for consent with full capacity, and use of the medication past the time of community supervision arise because it is assumed that sex offenders are likely to stop taking the medication when the opportunity arises. The side effects of feminization, common with long-term use of the antiandrogens and chemical castration, leading to failed reproductive capacity or consummation of relationships, are difficult to resolve.[26] Understanding relapse even with these medications or castration suggests that the benefit arising from the medications is appreciably measured and not risk-free or complete.

Resolving these ethical issues requires a good therapeutic relationship in which the risk-benefit ratio of the medications can be best analyzed and applied in management. When the goals of treatment include an offender's desires, safely incorporated in therapy, collaborative participation of that sort allows for the optimum use of pharmacologic agents. Those professionals trained in the medication and the prevention of adverse effects should be certified to treat sex offenders with medications.[12,28] Ongoing treatment in the hands of a novice clinician not only increases the chances of adverse consequences (prolongation of risk due to poor outcomes) but also may make rapport building more challenging in the future. The algorithm encompassing clinical guidelines for prescribers is a useful and practical step to managing and reducing these ethical risks.[12,27,28]

PSYCHOLOGICAL TREATMENT

The cornerstone for the treatment of sex offenders includes the development of an autobiographic account, creating a crime circle to understand the steps to offending, and proposing steps to prevent further reoffending based on identified risk factors. By recognizing the important risk-elevating factors, an offender can, with identified supports, monitor and modify them. Models with an evidence base, such as the good life model and approved sex offender treatment programs (SOTPs), are adopted with minor resource-related modifications.[22,29] With such models comes the value of the integrity of the SOTP without which ethical questions arise of standard treatment and its influence on public safety. A reduced risk for recidivism is linked with the proper administration of an SOTP.[22] Cognitive competence is required for such an endeavor and both personal commitment and professional guidance are required.[30] As may occur in individual sessions or preferably in group sessions, the preferred model may conflict with patient preference. Overrepresentation of female therapists in what is essentially a male-dominant problem is interesting. Instances of boundary violations are common and ethically challenging.[5,31] Close proximity with caring staff members for a protracted period of time is fertile grounds for emergence of transference and countertransference encounters. Unmanaged, these portend an increased risk of ethical misconduct.[32,33]

Clinical supervision and integrity of the treatment model and program are courted as a panacea for the ethical issues in psychological treatment. Collusion with an offender by an attracted staff member portends a high risk to others. Regular in-depth review of the principles and procedures as they adhere to the intents of the program could place all on alert to be professional and respectful in the program. Measures should be in place to ensure accountability that the evidence-based goals are cherished over individual preferences.[32,33] Self-incrimination by a patient is not an aberration and should be encouraged in treatment as long as guidelines exist for dealing safely with it.

SOCIAL INTERVENTION

Sex offenders who return to the community face several hurdles. When communities know about an offender coming to reside locally, in accordance with the notification laws, community reaction not uncommonly has led to expulsion from the locality. Going underground is a potential outcome of such extrication. Unfortunately, this can result in an increased risk to the community. Results of outcomes from the laws that contribute to this have been mixed.[34] Registration under a sex offender registry act, required by some if not most jurisdictions, can be protracted or a source of future offenses if a sex offender neglects to register. The ethical issue of infringement of the right to live as a free member of society is a real one.[3,7,26,34] An absence of supervision may cause persons to be vulnerable and the offenders, by restrictions to certain parts of society like schools and parks, to endure more discrimination. Those with the need to be in contact with young persons require the supervision of an adult. Employment opportunities are restricted once released to the community so support is needed to ensure recovery is not short chained. Although civil libertarians have decried the seemingly draconian steps toward managing sex offenders in the community as restricting and counter to safety, changing them requires directing efforts toward education and primary prevention measures.

Primary prevention requires self-recognition as a paraphiliac and allows a person, preferably an adolescent, to come forward willingly before offending starts. Such efforts will help resolve the dilemma that follows secretive offending under the disguise or fear that revelation will lead to prosecution. Educating the public about the rates of recidivism among sex offenders and strategies of minimizing victimization will likely improve the trust in and reliance on treatment programs that expect offenders to imbibe approaches that lead to risk reduction.[5,32] Much advancement in treatment and recidivism prevention is to be embraced and not feared.

STAGE OF COMMUNITY DISPOSITION AND RELAPSE

Commitment of sex offenders to a treatment plan postincarceration needs constant review and re-engagement. This is especially relevant when managing risk in the community matters a great deal. Policies, including civil commitment, community notification, sex offender registration, and mandatory community-based treatment, should be sufficient to fulfill rehabilitative goals of offenders as well as guarantee safety of the public. These policies have ethical drawbacks. Resolving ethical issues requires an adequate balancing of various needs, chief among them the best interests of offenders. Professionals should acknowledge the potential for coercion especially in court-ordered treatment or even in postadjudication cases.

Understanding involuntary treatment of some sex offenders can be assisted by parallel treatment obtained in mental health involuntary treatment and, in some jurisdictions, compulsory treatment of substance use disorder with or without complicating mental health symptoms. The common thread in these treatment approaches is the recognition of illness—impairment of help-seeking usually as a direct consequence of the illness, especially when adverse consequences are the natural outcome of the disorder. Also, efforts should be directed at keeping patients engaged in the relevant aspects of treatment.

Attrition from treatment is strongly associated with relapse.[5,22,32,35] Such knowledge behooves that attempts be directed at matching each deficit in an offender with the learning styles of that offender.[22,23] Adherence to the risk, need, and responsivity principles is proposed as a panacea to these difficulties. Evidence today points to a combination of regular communication, intensive supervision, and community treatment as the important step for reducing recidivism.[36] Use of an appropriate risk assessment measure to determine those who fail on supervision is again a highly contested ethical topic. This is prominent when norms are absent for individuals being assessed. Ethnic, cultural, and cognitive differences are central to the discussion.

RESEARCH

Research in the process, content, and outcome of sex offender treatment is ongoing and supported by public funds.[23,28] Procedures put in place to allow ethically guided research require supervision by higher authorities. Inducements to such a vulnerable population should be viewed carefully in accordance to current guidelines for research with human subjects. Research conducted through implied consent by attending a treatment program is ethically misguided, and retrospective data analyses have their ethical shortcomings. A full and informed consent should be the basis for research directed at answering practical issues rather than esoteric interests of researchers. Respect for autonomy is central to appropriate research activities.

SUMMARY

Every stage of involvement with sex offenders seeking treatment or mandated to take treatment is riddled with important ethical issues. Determining how to classify an offender, respect an offender's autonomy, and protect the public is premised on the conceptualization of the problem. From the perspective of disordered behaviors, treatment is carved out. To ensure permissible right and wrong behavior and conduct in dealing with a vulnerable population, such as those who mostly have been victimized and now victimize others, requires professionals certified and trained to navigate the conflicts inherent with managing them in and out of the treatment centers. The codes of conduct prescribed by professional bodies representing interventionists who work with sex offenders require dynamic updating and supervision. The goals of treatment and public safety when apposed closely help guide interactions between treatment staff and sex offenders. Realizing and applying the relevant values and safeguards are imperative to success.

REFERENCES

1. Huber P. Safety and the second best: the hazards of public risk management in the courts. Columbia Law Rev 1985;85(2):277–337. http://dx.doi.org/10.2307/1122439.
2. Corey Rayburn Y. Civil commitment for sex offenders. Virtual Mentor 2013;15(10):873–7.
3. Ryan RM, Deci EL. Intrinsic and extrinsic motivations: classic definitions and new directions. Contemp Educ Psychol 2000;25(1):54–67. http://dx.doi.org/10.1006/ceps.1999.1020.
4. Glaser B. Therapeutic jurisprudence: an ethical paradigm for therapists in sex offender treatment programs. West Crim Rev 2002;4:143.

5. Levenson J, D'Amora D. An ethical paradigm for sex offender treatment: response to Glaser. West Crim Rev 2005;6(1):145–53.

6. Birgden A, Cucolo H. The treatment of sex offenders: evidence, ethics, and human rights. Sex Abuse 2011;23(3):295–313. http://dx.doi.org/10.1177/1079063210381412.

7. Ward T, Rose C. Punishment and the Rehabilitation of Sex Offenders. In: Harrison K, Rainey B, editors. The Wiley-Blackwell Handbook of Legal and Ethical Aspects of Sex Offender Treatment and Management. Chichester, UK: John Wiley & Sons, Ltd; 2013. http://dx.doi.org/10.1002/9781118314876.ch16.

8. Falk AJ. Sex offenders, mental illness and criminal responsibility: the constitutional boundaries of civil commitment after Kansas v. Hendricks. Am J Law Med 1999;25:117.

9. Wakefield JC. DSM-5 proposed diagnostic criteria for sexual paraphilias: tensions between diagnostic validity and forensic utility [review]. Int J Law Psychiatry 2011;34(3):195–209.

10. McDougall J. Identifications, neoneeds and neosexualities [Case Reports]. Int J Psychoanal 1986;67(Pt 1):19–31.

11. Hill A, Habermann N, Berner W, et al. Sexual sadism and sadistic personality disorder in sexual homicide [Comparative Study Research Support, Non-U S Gov't]. J Pers Disord 2006;20(6):671–84.

12. Thibaut F. Pharmacological treatment of paraphilias. Isr J Psychiatry Relat Sci 2012;49(4):297–305.

13. Glaser B. Treaters or punishers? The ethical role of mental health clinicians in sex offender programs. Aggress Violent Behav 2009;14(4):248–55.

14. Serin RC, Mailloux DL. Assessment of sex offenders. Ann N Y Acad Sci 2003; 989(1):185–97. http://dx.doi.org/10.1111/j.1749-6632.2003.tb07305.x.

15. O'Shaughnessy R, Glancy G, Bradford J. Canadian landmark case, Smith v. Jones, supreme court of Canada: confidentiality and privilege suffer another blow. J Am Acad Psychiatry Law 1999;27(4):614–20.

16. Bonnar-Kidd KK. Sexual offender laws and prevention of sexual violence or recidivism. Am J Public Health 2010;100(3):412–9.

17. Card RD, Olsen SE. Visual plethysmograph stimuli involving children: rethinking some quasi-logical issues. Sex Abuse 1996;8(4):267–71. http://dx.doi.org/10.1177/107906329600800402.

18. Howes RJ. A survey of plethysmographic assessment in North America. Sex Abuse 1995;7(1):9–24. http://dx.doi.org/10.1177/107906329500700104.

19. Renaud P, Rouleau JL, Granger L, et al. Measuring sexual preferences in virtual reality: a pilot study [Research Support, Non-U.S. Gov't]. Cyberpsychol Behav 2002;5(1):1–9.

20. Agyapong VI, Kirrane R, Bangaru R. Medical confidentiality versus disclosure: ethical and legal dilemmas [Case Reports]. J Forensic Leg Med 2009;16(2):93–6.

21. Wijkman M, Bijleveld C, Hendriks J. Women don't do such things! Characteristics of female sex offenders and offender types. Sex Abuse 2010;22(2):135–56. http://dx.doi.org/10.1177/1079063210363826.

22. Olver ME, Wong SC, Nicholaichuk TP. Outcome evaluation of a high-intensity inpatient sex offender treatment program. J Interpers Violence 2009;24(3): 522–36. http://dx.doi.org/10.1177/0886260508317196.

23. McGrath RJ, Cumming GF, Hoke SE, et al. Outcomes in a community sex offender treatment program: a comparison between polygraphed and matched non-polygraphed offenders. Sex Abuse 2007;19(4):381–93. http://dx.doi.org/10.1177/107906320701900404.

24. Grisso T, Appelbaum PS. Assessing competence to consent to treatment: A guide for physicians and other health professionals. Oxford University Press; 1998.

25. Weinberger LE, Sreenivasan S, Garrick T, et al. The impact of surgical castration on sexual recidivism risk among sexually violent predatory offenders [Historical Article]. J Am Acad Psychiatry Law 2005;33(1):16–36.

26. Scott CL, Holmberg T. Castration of sex offenders: prisoners' rights versus public safety [review]. J Am Acad Psychiatry Law 2003;31(4):502–9.

27. Bradford JM. The neurobiology, neuropharmacology, and pharmacological treatment of the paraphilias and compulsive sexual behaviour. Can J Psychiatry 2001; 46(1):26–34.

28. Thibaut F, De La Barra F, Gordon H, et al. The World Federation of Societies of Biological Psychiatry (WFSBP) guidelines for the biological treatment of paraphilias [Practice Guideline]. World J Biol Psychiatry 2010;11(4):604–55. http://dx.doi.org/10.3109/15622971003671628.

29. Ward T, Gannon TA. Rehabilitation, etiology, and self-regulation: the comprehensive good lives model of treatment for sexual offenders. Aggress Violent Behav 2006;11(1):77–94. http://dx.doi.org/10.1016/j.avb.2005.06.001.

30. Scheela RA. Sex offender treatment: therapists' experiences and perceptions [Research Support, Non-U S Gov't]. Issues Ment Health Nurs 2001;22(8):749–67.

31. Schafer P, Peternelj-Taylor C. Therapeutic relationships and boundary maintenance: the perspective of forensic patients enrolled in a treatment program for violent offenders. Issues Ment Health Nurs 2003;24(6–7):605–25. http://dx.doi.org/10.1080/01612840305320.

32. Marshall WL, Ward T, Mann RE, et al. Working positively with sexual offenders: maximizing the effectiveness of treatment [review]. J Interpers Violence 2005; 20(9):1096–114.

33. Sarkar SP. Boundary violation and sexual exploitation in psychiatry and psychotherapy: a review. Adv Psychiatr Treat 2004;10(4):312–20. http://dx.doi.org/10.1192/apt.10.4.312.

34. Elbogen EB, Patry M, Scalora MJ. The impact of community notification laws on sex offender treatment attitudes. Int J Law Psychiatry 2003;26(2):207–19.

35. Parhar KK, Wormith JS, Derkzen DM, et al. Offender coercion in treatment: a meta-analysis of effectiveness. Crim Justice Behav 2008;35(9):1109–35. http://dx.doi.org/10.1177/0093854808320169.

36. Makarios MD, Latessa EJ. Intensive supervision programs: does program philosophy and the principles of effective intervention matter? J Crim Justice 2010;38: 368–75.

Index

Note: Page numbers of article titles are in **boldface** type.

A

Androgen-deprivation therapy, for paraphilic disorders, 177–178

Anxiety disorders, in mentaly disordered sexual offenders, obssessive compulsive disorder, 190

    social phobia and, 190

    types of, 189

Attention-deficit/hyperactivity disorder (ADHD), in mentaly disordered sexual offenders, group therapy for, 190–191

B

Behavior therapy, for child pornography offender, 209–210

C

Child pornography use, **207–214**

    assessment of, self-report in, 208

    management goals for, age and, 209

        gender of user and, 209

        psychiatric comorbidity and, 209

        vs. treatment, 209

    motivations for, 208

    nature of problem, 207–208

    prevention of, 212

    recommendations for, long term, 211

    treatment of, adjustment in, 211

        behavioral therapy in, 209–210

        Good Lives Model principles in, 210

        Internet Sex Offender Treatment Program, 210–211

        outcome evaluation of, 211

        self-management strategies in, 210–211

    types of users, pedophiles, 208

        sexually compulsive or hypersexual persons, 208, 212

Cognitive behavioral therapy, for sex offenders, 165–166, 225

Compliance with treatment, in persons with intellectual disabilities and problematic sexual behaviors, 202–203

Confidentiality, circle of in treatment, 244

Counterfit deviance, 197

Cyproterone acetate (CPA), contraindications to, 178

    informed consent for, 178

    uses of, 177–178

Psychiatr Clin N Am 37 (2014) 251–256
http://dx.doi.org/10.1016/S0193-953X(14)00043-4
0193-953X/14/$ – see front matter © 2014 Elsevier Inc. All rights reserved.

psych.theclinics.com

Moving?

Make sure your subscription moves with you!

To notify us of your new address, find your **Clinics Account Number** (located on your mailing label above your name), and contact customer service at:

Email: journalscustomerservice-usa@elsevier.com

800-654-2452 (subscribers in the U.S. & Canada)
314-447-8871 (subscribers outside of the U.S. & Canada)

Fax number: 314-447-8029

Elsevier Health Sciences Division
Subscription Customer Service
3251 Riverport Lane
Maryland Heights, MO 63043

*To ensure uninterrupted delivery of your subscription, please notify us at least 4 weeks in advance of move.

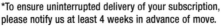

Printed and bound by CPI Group (UK) Ltd, Croydon, CR0 4YY

03/10/2024

01040489-0013